THE EMERGING FIELD OF HUMAN NEURAL ORGANOIDS, TRANSPLANTS, AND CHIMERAS

SCIENCE, ETHICS, AND GOVERNANCE

Committee on Ethical, Legal, and Regulatory Issues Associated with Neural Chimeras and Organoids

Committee on Science, Technology, and Law

Policy and Global Affairs

A Consensus Study Report of

The National Academies of
SCIENCES · ENGINEERING · MEDICINE

THE NATIONAL ACADEMIES PRESS
Washington, DC
www.nap.edu

THE NATIONAL ACADEMIES PRESS   500 Fifth Street, NW   Washington, DC 20001

This activity was supported by contracts from the National Institutes of Health (Sponsor Award Number HHSN263201800029I/75N98019F00861) and The Dana Foundation. This Project has been funded in whole or in part with federal funds from the National Institutes of Health, Department of Health and Human Services, under Contract No. HHSN263201800029I. Any opinions, findings, conclusions, or recommendations expressed in this publication do not necessarily reflect the views of any organization or agency that provided support for the project.

International Standard Book Number-13: 978-0-309-30336-1
International Standard Book Number-10: 0-309-30336-2
Digital Object Identifier: https://doi.org/10.17226/26078
Library of Congress Control Number: 2021938584

Cover image: High-magnification view of a neural organoid modeling early stages of development of the cerebral cortex. Image courtesy of Silvia Velasco and Paola Arlotta, Department of Stem Cell and Regenerative Biology, Harvard University.

Additional copies of this publication are available from the National Academies Press, 500 Fifth Street, NW, Keck 360, Washington, DC 20001; (800) 624-6242 or (202) 334-3313; http://www.nap.edu.

Copyright 2021 by the National Academy of Sciences. All rights reserved.

Printed in the United States of America

Suggested citation: National Academies of Sciences, Engineering, and Medicine. 2021. *The Emerging Field of Human Neural Organoids, Transplants, and Chimeras: Science, Ethics, and Governance.* Washington, DC: The National Academies Press. https://doi.org/10.17226/26078.

The National Academies of
SCIENCES • ENGINEERING • MEDICINE

The **National Academy of Sciences** was established in 1863 by an Act of Congress, signed by President Lincoln, as a private, nongovernmental institution to advise the nation on issues related to science and technology. Members are elected by their peers for outstanding contributions to research. Dr. Marcia McNutt is president.

The **National Academy of Engineering** was established in 1964 under the charter of the National Academy of Sciences to bring the practices of engineering to advising the nation. Members are elected by their peers for extraordinary contributions to engineering. Dr. John L. Anderson is president.

The **National Academy of Medicine** (formerly the Institute of Medicine) was established in 1970 under the charter of the National Academy of Sciences to advise the nation on medical and health issues. Members are elected by their peers for distinguished contributions to medicine and health. Dr. Victor J. Dzau is president.

The three Academies work together as the **National Academies of Sciences, Engineering, and Medicine** to provide independent, objective analysis and advice to the nation and conduct other activities to solve complex problems and inform public policy decisions. The National Academies also encourage education and research, recognize outstanding contributions to knowledge, and increase public understanding in matters of science, engineering, and medicine.

Learn more about the National Academies of Sciences, Engineering, and Medicine at **www.nationalacademies.org**.

The National Academies of
SCIENCES • ENGINEERING • MEDICINE

Consensus Study Reports published by the National Academies of Sciences, Engineering, and Medicine document the evidence-based consensus on the study's statement of task by an authoring committee of experts. Reports typically include findings, conclusions, and recommendations based on information gathered by the committee and the committee's deliberations. Each report has been subjected to a rigorous and independent peer-review process and it represents the position of the National Academies on the statement of task.

Proceedings published by the National Academies of Sciences, Engineering, and Medicine chronicle the presentations and discussions at a workshop, symposium, or other event convened by the National Academies. The statements and opinions contained in proceedings are those of the participants and are not endorsed by other participants, the planning committee, or the National Academies.

For information about other products and activities of the National Academies, please visit www.nationalacademies.org/about/whatwedo.

COMMITTEE ON ETHICAL, LEGAL, AND REGULATORY ISSUES ASSOCIATED WITH NEURAL CHIMERAS AND ORGANOIDS

Co-chairs

BERNARD LO (NAM), Professor Emeritus, University of California, San Francisco and President and CEO Emeritus, The Greenwall Foundation.
JOSHUA R. SANES (NAS), Jeff C. Tarr Professor of Molecular and Cellular Biology and Paul J. Finnegan Family Director, Center for Brain Science, Harvard University

Members

PAOLA ARLOTTA, Chair, Harvard Department of Stem Cell and Regenerative Biology and Golub Family Professor of Stem Cell and Regenerative Biology, Harvard University
R. ALTA CHARO (NAM), Warren P. Knowles Professor Emerita of Law and Bioethics, University of Wisconsin Law School
JOHN H. EVANS, Professor, Tata Chancellor's Chair in Social Sciences, Associate Dean of Social Sciences, and Co-director of the Institute for Practical Ethics, University of California, San Diego
FRED H. GAGE (NAS/NAM), President and Professor, Laboratory of Genetics, and Vi and John Adler Chair for Research on Age-Related Neurodegenerative Disease, Salk Institute for Biological Studies
HENRY T. GREELY, Deane F. and Kate Edelman Johnson Professor of Law, Professor, by courtesy, of Genetics, Stanford School of Medicine, and Director, Center for Law and the Biosciences, Stanford University
PATRICIA A. KING (NAM), Professor Emerita, Georgetown University Law Center
WILLIAM T. NEWSOME (NAS), Harman Family Provostial Professor of Neurobiology, Stanford University School of Medicine, and Vincent V.C. Woo Director, Wu Tsai Neurosciences Institute, Stanford University
SALLY TEMPLE, Scientific Director, Principal Investigator, and Co-Founder, Neural Stem Cell Institute
A. LAWRENCE ZIPURSKY (NAS), Distinguished Professor, Department of Biological Chemistry, University of California, Los Angeles, and Investigator, Howard Hughes Medical Institute

Staff

ANNE-MARIE MAZZA, Study Director and Senior Director, Committee on Science, Technology, and Law
STEVEN KENDALL, Program Officer, Committee on Science, Technology, and Law

ANITA EISENSTADT, Program Officer, U.S. Science and Innovation Policy
VERN DUNN, Program Officer, U.S. Science and Innovation Policy
DOMINIC LOBUGLIO, Senior Program Assistant, Committee on Science, Technology, and Law
SARAH CARTER, Consultant Writer

COMMITTEE ON SCIENCE, TECHNOLOGY, AND LAW

Co-Chairs

DAVID BALTIMORE (NAS/NAM), President Emeritus and Robert Andrews Millikan Professor of Biology, California Institute of Technology
DAVID S. TATEL, Judge, U.S. Court of Appeals for the District of Columbia Circuit

Members

JOE S. CECIL, Senior Fellow, Civil Justice Research Initiative, University of California, Berkeley School of Law
ERWIN CHEMERINSKY, Dean and Jesse H. Choper Distinguished Professor, University of California, Berkeley School of Law
ELLEN WRIGHT CLAYTON (NAM), Professor of Law and Professor of Health Policy, Vanderbilt University Medical Center
JOHN S. COOKE, Director, Federal Judicial Center
JOHN DABIRI, Centennial Professor of Aeronautics and Mechanical Engineering, California Institute of Technology
JENNIFER EBERHARDT (NAS), Professor of Psychology, Stanford University
FEI-FEI LI (NAE/NAM), Sequoia Capital Professor, by courtesy, of Operations, Information and Technology, Stanford University
JUDITH MILLER, Independent Consultant
MARTHA MINOW, 300th Anniversary University Professor, Harvard Law School
KIMANI PAUL-EMILE, Professor of Law, Fordham University Law School
NATALIE RAM, Associate Professor of Law, University of Maryland Francis King Carey School of Law
LISA RANDALL (NAS), Professor of Theoretical Physics, Harvard University
PAUL M. ROMER, Professor of Economics and Director, The Urbanization Project, New York University
WILLIAM B. SCHULTZ, Partner, Zuckerman Spaeder LLP
JOSHUA SHARFSTEIN (NAM), Vice Dean and Professor, Johns Hopkins Bloomberg School of Public Health
SUSAN S. SILBEY, Leon and Anne Goldberg Professor of Humanities, Professor of Sociology and Anthropology, and Professor of Behavioral and Policy Sciences, Massachusetts Institute of Technology
SRI SRINIVASAN, Chief Judge, U.S. Court of Appeals for the District of Columbia Circuit
GREGORY STONE, Partner, Munger, Tolles & Olson LLP
SUSAN WESSLER (NAS), Neil and Rochelle Campbell Presidential Chair for Innovation in Science Education, University of California, Riverside, and Home Secretary, U.S. National Academy of Sciences

Staff

ANNE-MARIE MAZZA, Senior Director
STEVEN KENDALL, Program Officer
DOMINIC LOBUGLIO, Senior Program Associate

Preface

More than any other organ, the brain gives human beings their unique identities. The complexity of the human brain has perplexed researchers, and its central role in the mystery termed consciousness continues to challenge the boundaries between science and philosophy. Conversely, devastating neurological and psychiatric diseases and disorders not only cause untold suffering but can also rob people of their identity. For many of these diseases, treatments are completely unavailable, and for others they are hopelessly inadequate.

Research over the past several decades has greatly advanced understanding of the brain and begun to provide new therapeutic approaches to brain diseases. However, progress in this area is stymied by the practical and ethical difficulties of studying the human brain and by serious limitations of existing tools and models. In response, researchers have worked to develop new models that promise a deeper understanding of the human brain and new treatments for brain disorders. These new models include human neural organoids, transplants of human stem cells into nonhuman animal brains, and human neural chimeras. However, as models of the brain improve to better reflect the characteristics of actual human brains, they also raise profound ethical questions. It has become clear that in using these models to advance understanding of the brain, it will be necessary to pay attention to what lessons they might teach about consciousness and what it means to be human.

For the past year, at the request of the National Institutes of Health and the Dana Foundation and under the auspices of the National Academies of Sciences, Engineering, and Medicine's Committee on Science, Technology, and Law, we co-chaired a committee of scientists, ethicists, and legal scholars that explored recent scientific advances and ethical and governance issues associated with human neural organoids, transplants, and chimeras. The committee heard from numerous experts and reviewed relevant scientific literature, religious scholarship, and current laws and policies. We are grateful for the individuals who spoke to and engaged in thoughtful discussions with the committee. Their expertise contributed greatly to the committee's deliberations. In particular, interactions among biomedical scientists, ethicists, religious scholars, and legal experts provided the committee with important insights.

We are deeply indebted to the committee members for the time and effort they devoted to reading and reviewing background materials; preparing for discussions with invited experts; attending virtual meetings; and engaging in thoughtful, critical analysis and discussion with each other. This report is a reflection of their commitment to understanding the issues under consideration.

We greatly appreciate as well the efforts of study director Anne-Marie Mazza and study staff Steven Kendall, Anita Eisenstadt, Vern Dunn, and Dominic LoBuglio and of consultant writer, Sarah Carter.

Bernard Lo and Joshua R. Sanes,
Committee co-chairs

Acknowledgments

Acknowledgment of Presenters

The committee gratefully acknowledges the thoughtful contributions of the following individuals who made presentations before the committee:

Megan Albertelli, Stanford University; Mark Barnes, Ropes & Gray LLP; Allan Basbaum (NAS/NAM), University of California, San Francisco; Valerie Bonham, Ropes & Gray LLP; Emery Brown (NAS/NAM/NAE), Massachusetts Institute of Technology; I. Glenn Cohen, Harvard Law School; Charles Camosy, Fordham University; David DeGrazia, George Washington University; Frans B. M. de Waal, Emory University; Brian Edlow, Massachusetts General Hospital; Nita Farahany, Duke University School of Law; Guoping Feng, Massachusetts Institute of Technology; Steven Goldman, University of Rochester Medical Center; Steven E. Hyman (NAM), Harvard University and Dana Foundation; Insoo Hyun, Case Western Reserve University; Eva Jablonka, Tel-Aviv University; Kathleen Hall Jamieson (NAS), University of Pennsylvania; Christof Koch, Allen Institute for Brain Science; Arnold Kriegstein (NAM), University of California, San Francisco; Margaret Landi, GlaxoSmithKline; John Loike, Columbia University; Robin Lovell-Badge, The Francis Crick Institute; Brad Margus, Cerevance; Sergiu Pasca, Stanford University; James Peterson, Roanoke College; Mu-Ming Poo (NAS), Institute of Neuroscience of the Chinese Academy of Sciences; Margaret Foster Riley, University of Virginia School of Law; Dietram Scheufele, University of Wisconsin–Madison; Bjoern Schwer, University of California, San Francisco; Anil Seth, University of Sussex; Sarra Tlili, University of Florida; Joyce Tischler, Lewis & Clark Law School; Gordana Vunjak-Novakovic (NAE/NAM), Columbia University; and Carrie Wolinetz, National Institutes of Health.

Acknowledgment of Reviewers

This Consensus Study Report was reviewed in draft form by individuals chosen for their diverse perspectives and technical expertise. The purpose of this independent review is to provide candid and critical comments that will assist the National Academies of Sciences, Engineering, and Medicine in making each published report as sound as possible and to ensure that it meets the institutional standards for quality, objectivity, evidence, and responsiveness to the study charge. The review comments and draft manuscript remain confidential to protect the integrity of the deliberative process.

We thank the following individuals for their review of this report:

Charles Camosy, Fordham University; Patricia Churchland, University of California, San Diego; Ellen Wright Clayton (NAM), Vanderbilt University; I. Glenn Cohen, Harvard University; Jonathan Flint, University of California, Los Angeles; Michael Goldberg (NAS), Columbia University; Steven Goldman, University of Rochester Medical Center; Gillian Hue, Emory University; Insoo Hyun, Case Western Reserve University; Madeline Lancaster, University of Cambridge; Margaret Landi, GlaxoSmithKline; James Peterson, Roanoke College; Alex Pollen, University of California, San Francisco; Anil Seth, University of Sussex; Hongjun Song (NAM), University of Pennsylvania; and Robert Streiffer, University of Wisconsin–Madison.

Although the reviewers listed above provided many constructive comments and suggestions, they were not asked to endorse the conclusions or recommendations of this report nor did they see the final draft before its release. The review of this report was overseen by Wylie Burke (NAM), University of Washington, and Thomas D. Albright (NAS), Salk Institute for Biological Studies. They were responsible for making certain that an independent examination of this report was carried out in accordance with the standards of the National Academies and that all review comments were carefully considered. Responsibility for the final content rests entirely with the authoring committee and the National Academies.

Table of Contents

SUMMARY   1

1   INTRODUCTION   11
    Overview of Brain Research, 12
    Study Charge, 14
    Organization of the Report, 16

2   THE SCIENCE OF HUMAN NEURAL ORGANOIDS,
    TRANSPLANTS, AND CHIMERAS   19
    Human Neural Organoids, 26
    Human Neural Transplants, 31
    Human Neural Chimeras, 32
    Capacities of Human Neural Organoids, Transplants, and Chimeras, 34
    Measuring Characteristics of Human Neural Organoids, Transplants,
        and Chimeras, 41

3   ETHICAL CONCERNS   45
    Issues Common to All Three Models, 46
    Issues Specific to Human Neural Organoids, Transplants,
        and Chimeras, 52
    Ethical Issues Specific to Human Neural Organoids, 63
    Summary, 64

4   OVERSIGHT AND GOVERNANCE   65
    Use of Human Stem Cells, 66

Informed Consent, 69
Use and Care of Animals in Research, 72
Use of Nonhuman Primates in Research, 74
U.S. Policy and Guidance Specific to Neural Transplants
    and Chimeras, 75
Graded Oversight: A Three-Tiered Approach, 82
International Policy Specific to Neural Organoids, Transplants,
    and Chimeras, 82
Future Oversight, 86

5   PUBLIC ENGAGEMENT   91
    Public Engagement Internationally and in the United States, 91
    Potential Contribution of Social Science Research, 93
    Nomenclature, 94

6   FINDINGS OF THE COMMITTEE   97
    Value of This Research, 97

REFERENCES   105

APPENDIXES

A   Biographies of Committee and Staff Members   119
B   Committee Meeting Agendas   129

Boxes, Figures, and Tables

BOXES

2-1 The Nervous System, 20

4-1 Illustrative Oversight Scenarios, 80

FIGURES

1-1 Human neural organoids and assembloids, 13
1-2 Human neural transplants and chimeras, 15

2-1 Architecture of the human nervous system, 24
2-2 Cells of the nervous system, 25
2-3 Embryonic stem cells (ESCs) and induced pluripotent stem cells (iPSCs), 27
2-4 Use of induced pluripotent stem cells (iPSCs) to analyze mechanisms of brain disease, 29
2-5 Distinct evolutionary views of consciousness, 38

TABLES

3-1 The Three R's, 58

4-1 Oversight of Research Based on the Use of Human Stem Cells, 68
4-2 Oversight of Research on Human Neural Cell Transplants and Neural Chimeras, 76

4-3 Examples of Human Neural Organoid, Transplant, and Chimera Research Subject to Different Levels of Scrutiny, 83

Summary[1]

Each year, tens of millions of individuals in the United States suffer from neurological and psychiatric disorders, including neurodegenerative diseases such as Alzheimer's disease and Parkinson's disease, and psychiatric disorders such as autism spectrum disorder, depression, and schizophrenia. Treatments for these diseases are often completely lacking or only partially effective. The dearth of treatments is due in large part to the difficulty of conducting research on an organ containing nearly 100 billion neurons interconnected by trillions of synaptic connections in intricate circuits that can hold vast amounts of information. Unsurprisingly, such complexity presents formidable challenges, and tools for studying complex circuits typical of the brain are limited. Additionally, there is a lack of good experimental systems for testing disease mechanisms and therapies. While animal models used to study brain structure and function have been indispensable, there are key molecular, cellular, and structural differences between the brains of rodents or even nonhuman primates and those of humans. These shortcomings may help explain why disease treatments that have shown promise in animal models are often ineffective in humans.

Over the past few decades, scientific advances have yielded greater understanding of how neurons develop, function, connect, and underlie some simple behaviors. These advances have positioned brain researchers to use this knowledge to tackle human disease mechanisms and design effective therapies. However, making this leap is difficult largely because of the many ethical, legal, and practical limitations to studying the human brain. To address some of these limita-

---

[1] This summary does not include references. Sources for the information herein are cited in the main text of the report.

tions, researchers in recent years have developed new models to better represent and study the human brain. The three models considered in this report—all of which exploit the ability to generate and use pluripotent stem cells from individual humans or human embryos—are human neural organoids, human neural cell transplants (sometimes called xenografts), and human neural chimeras.

- *Human neural organoids* are three-dimensional aggregates of human neural cells grown in the laboratory from stem cells. While small (currently no more than 4mm in diameter), neural organoids recapitulate some important features of fetal human brains, exhibiting, for example, key developmental, cellular, and molecular characteristics. Current neural organoids are limited in complexity and maturity, but researchers are working to overcome these limitations.
- *Human neural transplants*[2] are generated by transplanting human cells into the brains of model organisms, under conditions that favor their differentiation into neurons or glia. Human cells have been transplanted into nonhuman animals for decades, with the use of stem cells for transplantation a more recent advance. These transplants enable the study of human neurons, glia, and other brain cells in the context of a whole, behaving organism. Moreover, human neurons, glia, and other cells have already been transplanted into the adult human nervous system as a potential therapy for neurodegenerative disease. Transplantation into nonhuman animals can provide preclinical data essential for designing these and other new therapies.
- *Human neural chimeras* are a special case of transplants. To generate a chimera, stem cells are injected into a nonhuman host very early in embryonic development. They then intermingle with the host cells that form the brain, populating it from the earliest stage and developing in parallel with the host. In one variant of the method, called blastocyst complementation, the transplanted stem cells replace most of the host cells in a particular brain region. To date, chimeras that develop to fetal stages or later have been generated only using rodent stem cells placed in rodent hosts. Research in this area is advancing rapidly, however, and it is possible that chimeras could be generated from human cells injected into the blastocyst of a nonhuman primate. These methods will not be applicable to humans as therapies, but their potential as a research model is great.

Human neural organoids, cell transplants, and chimeras are already yielding important insights into the functioning of the human brain and human brain

---

[2] In this report, human neural transplant refers to the transplantation of human neural cells or groups of human neural cells into the brains of nonhuman animals. The transplantation of large portions of the human brain has not been proposed to date and is currently infeasible. Such transplants are excluded from consideration in this report.

disorders. As they become more like real human brains and improve as model systems, however, they raise difficult ethical questions: As human brain organoids become larger and more complex, could they acquire aspects of consciousness? Could they "feel" pain? As scientists successfully integrate more human cells into the brains of transplanted and chimeric animals, could the resulting animal have capacities substantially different from those typical of their species? If so, would they need to be treated differently than other laboratory animals? Do chimeras violate the distinction between humans and other animals that is deeply embedded in many cultures? Could the animals develop characteristics that are commonly thought of as human?

STUDY CHARGE

This report, funded by the National Institutes of Health and the Dana Foundation, examines the state of human neural organoid, transplant, and chimera and neural organoid research, and considers whether there exist thresholds at which these model systems might become objects of greater moral concern. The committee convened by the National Academies of Sciences, Engineering, and Medicine to conduct this study was asked to review the status of this research, consider its benefits and risks, examine associated ethical issues, and consider what oversight mechanisms might be appropriate in this area. For this report, the sponsors directed that the committee provide consensus findings on these topics, but not make specific recommendations. The committee was asked to consider such questions as

- How would researchers define or identify enhanced or human awareness in a chimeric animal?
- Do research animals with enhanced capabilities require different treatment compared to typical animal models?
- What are appropriate disposal mechanisms for such models?
- What types of brain tissue are appropriate for use as neural organoids?
- How large or complex would the ex vivo brain organoids need to be to attain enhanced or human awareness?
- What kind of "humanized" brain, in size and structure, would be acceptable in a research animal?
- Should patients give explicit consent for their cells to be used to create neural organoids?
- What regulatory mechanisms relating to organoid and chimeric animal research are currently in place? Are there gaps in the current regulatory framework?
- What regulatory mechanisms exist for similar research?
- What further regulatory mechanisms might be appropriate?

Examination of these issues required both assessment of the relevant science and consideration of ethical and philosophical issues related to humanness, consciousness, self-awareness, and the welfare of entities with altered or "enhanced" capacities. To carry out these tasks, the committee conducted an extensive literature review and held seven virtual meetings in which experts provided diverse perspectives on neuroscience research, animal models, theories of consciousness, religious scholarship, ethics, animal welfare, and other relevant areas. After considerable discussion and analysis, the committee developed the findings detailed below to provide guidance for scientists, clinicians, regulators, and the general public as they consider how to balance the value of this research with the ethical concerns it raises.

STUDY FINDINGS

The committee's findings fall into six areas:

1. Value of this research
2. State of the science
3. Issues of ethical concern
4. Assessment of consciousness and pain in human neural organoids, transplants, and chimeras
5. Oversight and regulation
6. Public engagement and communication

Value of This Research

Finding I.1: Brain diseases—neurological and psychiatric disorders—are the leading cause of morbidity worldwide, resulting in mortality and untold suffering, as well as enormous financial burdens in health care costs and lost wages. There are few if any highly effective treatments for many of these disorders, which include traumatic injury; neurodegenerative diseases, such as Alzheimer's disease, Parkinson's disease, and amyotrophic lateral sclerosis; psychiatric diseases, such as schizophrenia and bipolar disorder; developmental disorders, such as autism spectrum disorder; and brain cancers. The lack of progress in developing therapeutics for these disorders in large part reflects a lack of knowledge regarding the underlying disease processes in the developing or adult brain and how brain aging contributes to disease onset and progression. The development of new therapies will require a foundation of greater basic knowledge about human brain development, maturation, and function and greater translational knowledge about the mechanisms of brain diseases. However, research on the human brain itself is limited by a combination of legal, practical, and ethical restrictions, as well as technical hurdles. Small animal models provide a valuable alternative, but they are insufficient for studying complex human brain disorders.

Finding I.2: Recent advances in human stem cell research now enable ready access to human neurons and glial cells, facilitating the development of more sophisticated models with which to study brain diseases and disorders in greater depth. Human neural organoids, transplants, and chimeras are powerful models that use stem cells to circumvent many of the limitations noted above, providing novel ways to understand normal and abnormal human brain development, analyze disease mechanisms, and assess therapeutic approaches. Thus, they have the potential to be invaluable additions to human studies and animal models. The promise of these novel human brain cell models is that they will contribute to understanding of the mechanisms of brain development and function, and pave the way for the development of transformative therapies that can relieve the significant burden of neurological and psychiatric diseases. However, this promise must be carefully weighed against the ethical concerns such models may raise.

State of the Science

Finding II.1: Human neural organoids are cellular aggregates derived from human stem cells, in which multiple, diverse types of neuronal and glial cells differentiate and form three-dimensional organized assemblies. They have been used to model several aspects of human brain development and structure. Organoids generated from patient-derived stem cells sometimes exhibit disease phenotypes that can be used to elucidate pathogenic mechanisms and test potential interventions. However, organoids are limited in size and complexity and lack important cell types, brain regions, and anatomically organized neural circuits thought to be required for complex human brain function, including consciousness. Researchers are actively pursuing new techniques for overcoming these limitations of organoids, and this work will likely lead to organoids of increased size and greater complexity. Maturation is also likely to be improved, but the likelihood of generating a structure with the intricate organization, wealth of diverse cell types, and complex interconnectedness that would resemble in any significant way the mature functioning human brain is remote for the foreseeable future.

Finding II.2: Transplantation of human neural cells into the brains of nonhuman animals shows promise for improving models of neurological and psychiatric disease. Human glial precursors can be introduced into the brain of animal models, where they differentiate, integrate, and function. However, limitations exist that determine the level of maturation and integration of the transplanted cells within the host brain. These limitations are due to species-specific differences in developmental times whereby, for example, human brain cells mature much more slowly than their mouse counterparts, even upon transplantation in the mouse brain. The result is a developmental mismatch that is likely to affect the contribution of human neural cells to the working circuits of the host.

In chimeric animals (as defined above), donor[3] and host cells develop together from the earliest stages of embryogenesis. In one such method, blastocyst complementation, host cells that would normally contribute to particular brain regions are eliminated at an early stage, allowing extensive replacement of those regions by donor cells. To date, neural chimeras generated by these methods use donor and host cells from the same or closely related species. It is not currently possible to generate neural chimeras of human cells in embryos of any nonhuman species that survive postnatally or even to late fetal stages. Generation of such chimeras may eventually be more feasible in nonhuman primates than in rodents.

Issues of Ethical Concern

Finding III.1: Because of the human suffering and mortality caused by brain disorders, limitations of current animal disease models, and the uniquely human quality of some brain diseases, there are strong moral arguments in favor of research using organoids, transplants, and chimeras derived from human cells as long as such research is balanced with other ethical considerations, such as ensuring animal welfare, appropriate use of human biological materials, and safety.

Finding III.2: Some studies in which human neural cells have been integrated into the brains of nonhuman animals raise moral, ethical, and religious concerns regarding the mixing of humans and other animals, the special status of humans, animals acquiring attributes that could be viewed as distinctively human, or humans taking on roles that should be reserved for a deity. Similar objections may also be raised from a secular viewpoint—for example, that conducting such research shows hubris or that the resulting entity offends the dignity of human beings.

A key concern is that a fundamental distinction between humans and other animals could be blurred. The increasing ability to generate human-animal chimeras with greater integration of human neural cells heightens this concern. There may also be concerns that some human cells outside the body should not be treated as mere clumps of matter. Some types of cells, such as human blastocysts and embryonic stem cells that are considered potential or actual human beings, are accorded greater or special respect, depending on one's religious and philosophical views.

Finding III.3: Under Subpart A of the Federal Policy for the Protection of Human Subjects, often called the Common Rule, existing biological materials that have been collected with appropriate consent and deidentified may be used in future research projects. However, provisions of the Common Rule are seen by some as a minimal standard for meeting ethical requirements in this area.

---

[3] In this report, a donor refers to the person from whom materials were obtained for derivation.

For biological materials collected in the past, specific consent for human neural organoid, transplant, and chimera research was generally not obtained. There is active discussion regarding the advantages and disadvantages of obtaining specific consent going forward for the collection of fresh tissue for such research.

As a practical matter, recontacting donors to obtain specific consent is sometimes impossible. Moreover, many induced pluripotent stem cell (iPSC) lines obtained from donor tissue have been extensively characterized or were derived from patients with very rare diseases, and deriving new lines would be extremely difficult in these cases. On the other hand, most donors were not aware that their tissues would be used for neural organoid, transplant, or chimera research, and some might have objected if directly asked for their consent for such uses. Past ethics violations during research with African American and Native American participants make this a sensitive topic for these populations.

Finding III.4: Nonhuman animals have interests and some believe they have rights. Humans should therefore respect their well-being and their intrinsic nature and telos. However, there is wide agreement that it is permissible to use animals for basic and translational research directed toward the goal of relieving human suffering as long as the research is justified in terms of prospective benefit to human health, harm to animals is minimized, and the needs of the animals are met. Well-established regulations and practices emphasize the requirements to minimize the number of animals used; replace them with other experimental models when possible and consistent with the approved scientific aims of the research; alleviate or minimize their pain and distress; and provide them appropriate living conditions, including nutritious food, safe shelter, housing, companionship, and opportunities for stimulation.

As transplantation and chimeric models of human brain diseases become better able to model key disease features, research animals are likely to show behaviors that resemble human symptoms and that would be viewed as distressing were they to occur in humans. Close observation of the animals can identify such behaviors, which may need to be avoided or mitigated to maintain animal welfare. Another concern is that host animals might acquire altered behaviors wholly atypical of their species, such as new forms of problem solving or substantially altered, complex social interactions. If so, objections to using such animals for research might increase. The committee found scant evidence that this is a realistic possibility in the foreseeable future, but surveillance of this rapidly developing research is essential.

Finding III.5: The complexity of neural organoids is currently limited. It is extremely unlikely that in the foreseeable future they would possess capacities that, given current understanding, would be recognized as awareness, consciousness, emotion, or the experience of pain. Thus, it appears at present that neural organoids have no more moral standing than other in vitro human neural tissues or cultures. As scientists develop significantly more complex organoids, however, the need to make this distinction will need to be revisited regularly. Moreover, organoids can be transplanted into the brain, blurring the distinction between organoids and transplants.

Assessment of Consciousness and Pain in Human Neural Organoids, Transplants, and Chimeras

Finding IV.1: Decisions about how research on neural cell transplantation and chimeras should be conducted or overseen depend in large part on the possibility that the animal host will have altered capacities as a consequence of its brain cells being augmented or replaced by human cells. The possibilities of pain sensation, and altered consciousness are often raised as issues of particular concern, but both pain and consciousness are difficult to define or measure. While measurements of neuronal activity and circuit physiology are possible in organoids, these measurements are not considered sufficient to determine whether organoids may be conscious or feel pain. In contrast, when human cells are incorporated in a host brain, via either chimera formation or cell transplantation, it will be possible to devise and deploy methods for detecting differences in the behavior of that host compared with that of a host in which human cells have not been integrated. Some metrics and indicators already exist, particularly for pain. Likewise, there are quantitative methods for assessing behavior with high temporal and spatial resolution. Research veterinarians, ethologists, and animal behavior researchers are well suited to providing guidance on how to identify and interpret behaviors that are not typical of the species or the individual.

Finding IV.2: Most current methods for assessing consciousness (sometimes called awareness or sentience) and pain cannot be applied to organoids because understanding of these capacities depends largely on observing behaviors in whole animals. With the current state of knowledge, it would be difficult to use these measurements as evidence for the existence of pain or consciousness in organoids.

Oversight and Regulation

Finding V.1: Many ethical concerns raised by current and near-future research can be addressed by current oversight mechanisms, which are often created for specific ethical purposes. Nonetheless, some concerns will need be reassessed as the science develops.

Finding V.2: Neural organoids will not raise issues that require additional oversight until and unless they become significantly more complex.

Finding V.3: Transplantation of human neural cells or human neural organoids into nonhuman animals falls under a well-developed oversight system for animal research. In the United States, this system is built on the Animal Welfare Act and the Public Health Service Policy on Humane Care and Use of Laboratory Animals (PHS Policy). It includes review and approval of research protocols by institutional animal care and use committees (IACUCs), as well as on-the-ground monitoring by research veterinarians and animal caregivers. As currently constituted, however, some IACUCs may not contain sufficient independent expertise in neural cell transplant or chimera research or interpretation of animal behavior after transplantation of human neural cells.

Finding V.4: The animal welfare concerns raised by the generation of neural chimeras through blastocyst complementation in rodents also fall under significant and capable oversight by IACUCs and research veterinarians. Again, however, additional expertise on topics such as behavioral capabilities may be required.

Finding V.5: Some future research, including that involving more complex human neural organoids, transplants, and chimeras and the generation of transplants and chimeras in nonhuman primates, will benefit from additional discussion of ethical and social issues that extend beyond reviews of individual research projects currently carried out by IACUCs. Examples include injection of human stem cells into nonhuman animal blastocysts and indications that suggest enhanced capacities in transplant recipients or chimeras. Possibilities for additional oversight or safeguards include pilot studies followed by re-evaluation, implementation of novel measures to monitor capacities of research animals, and designation of research that should not be conducted at this time. There are advantages to carrying out such discussions at the national level, where a wide range of viewpoints and disciplinary backgrounds could be convened.

Finding V.6: Interdisciplinary research organizations, such as the International Society for Stem Cell Research (ISSCR), periodically analyze the updated state of the science, but no national or governmental bodies in the United States have this task as part of their mandate. Moreover, there is currently no national body in the United States whose charge is to review emerging science in key areas or to assess their ethical and regulatory implications.

Finding V.7: In several fields of innovative and rapidly developing biomedical research that raise social and ethical concerns, such as human embryonic stem cell research and human genome editing, a three-tiered system of oversight has been recommended and, in some cases, adopted:

- research that can be carried out under current oversight procedures,
- research that requires heightened oversight, and
- research that should not be carried out at this time.

This system allows ethically uncontroversial research projects to be carried out without imposing an administrative burden while providing additional scrutiny of research projects for which attention to emergent issues or additional expertise in the review body is helpful.

Prohibition of some types of research can reflect widely accepted limits on research that have been articulated by public and scientific groups. A prohibition on conducting such research at present also allows for later reconsideration once the science has matured enough to understand its consequences, along with an updated assessment of ethical considerations.

Public Engagement and Communication

Finding VI.1: Calls have been increasing for greater public engagement in assessing the value of emerging areas of biomedical research. Such engagement has several benefits, including helping the public understand the research, identifying public concerns, facilitating informed public discussion, and influencing science policy. However, the United States currently lacks robust mechanisms for facilitating this public engagement. Analysis of lessons learned from efforts on related topics could support the design of effective strategies for engaging the public in discussion of human neural organoids, transplants, and chimeras.

Finding VI.2: Well-designed social science research could also help scientists, regulators, and policy makers better understand the views of the public. Social science research on public attitudes toward and perspectives on human neural organoid and chimera research is currently lacking in the United States.

Finding VI.3: During its meetings and deliberations, the committee appreciated hearing the perspectives of religious scholars of several faith traditions and engaging in discussions with experts in medicine, biology, philosophy, law, theology, religious studies, and other disciplines. These discussions were mutually enlightening and should be continued. Because of the plurality of religious and secular views in the United States, ongoing dialogues between religious and secular perspectives and among different viewpoints are important. There are currently few if any established forums for fostering this exchange.

Finding VI.4: In some cases, terms used to describe human neural organoids, transplants, and chimeras have been inaccurate, inadequately descriptive, or misleading. These terms can evoke, intentionally or unintentionally, emotional responses that do not reflect the science being described, and they can be used to pull the public toward acceptance or rejection of a technology. As one of many examples, neural organoids are often referred to in the press as "mini-brains," but in reality, they model only some limited aspects of brain tissue. Closer attention to issues of nomenclature by scientists and their institutional representatives in their interactions with the press and public would facilitate a more informed public debate about brain research.

1

Introduction

A major reason that researchers seek to understand the human brain is to prevent, treat, and cure neurological and psychiatric diseases. These diseases, which affect tens of millions each year (Disease and Injury Incidence and Prevalence Collaborators, 2018), include neurodegenerative diseases such as Alzheimer's disease and Parkinson's disease, and psychiatric disorders such as autism spectrum disorder, depression, and schizophrenia. Treatments for these conditions are partially effective at best and in some cases are completely lacking. In addition to the suffering and disability faced by affected individuals and their families, brain diseases have a tremendous economic impact. In 2017, neurological disorders were estimated to cost more than $800 billion per year in the United States, including costs related to both clinical care and lost productivity due to disability and mortality (Gooch et al., 2017). Psychiatric diseases take a similar toll, annually imposing total costs exceeding $200 billion in the United States (Greenberg et al., 2015) and reaching up to $2.5 trillion globally (Trautmann et al., 2016). Depression and anxiety disorders alone account for 8 percent of years lived with disability worldwide (Disease and Injury Incidence and Prevalence Collaborators, 2018). In this context, the National Institutes of Health (NIH) has made brain research a priority, budgeting over $10 billion in 2020 to improve our understanding of the brain and its disorders (NIH, 2020).

Given the devastating toll of brain diseases, there is strong public interest in research advances that offer hope for their treatment or cure. Furthermore, the brain captures the public imagination: Everyone understands that the brain defines human beings in fundamental ways. However, news reports and blog posts sometimes fail to satisfy this curiosity in appropriate ways. Rather, they may describe brain research in terms that maximize attention at the expense of scientific accuracy. Headlines regarding research described in this report include, for example, "Lab-Grown 'Mini Brains' Can Now Mimic the Neural Activity of a Preterm Infant" (Stetka, 2019), "Scientists Re-create Baby Brain Readings in a Dish" (Devlin, 2019; Fernandez, 2019; Grossman, 2018), "The smart mouse with the half-human brain" (Coghlan, 2014), and "These mice have brains that are part human. So are they mice, or men?" (Nogrady, 2018). These news articles draw from scientific publications and interviews with researchers and sometimes quote the scientists involved. Nonetheless, the implications are misleading—researchers are not currently developing miniature brains in a vat, and there are no mouse brains that are half human. These articles fuel uneasiness about brain research involving human neural organoids, transplants, and chimeras.

That is not to say, however, that uneasiness about such research is inappropriate. Most would agree with the statement, "If I receive your kidney as a transplant, I am still me, but if I receive your brain as a transplant, I'm not sure who I'd be." Therefore, research that involves human brain cells, despite its potential to provide new therapies for brain diseases, raises legitimate concerns about what is appropriate and whether it might result in the erosion of moral distinctions. This report begins by describing some of the advances achieved in these areas of research and then goes on to examine the ethical and societal concerns that they raise.

OVERVIEW OF BRAIN RESEARCH

Research on the brain is difficult, and advances in understanding of how the brain works have lagged progress in other biomedical fields. The human brain contains nearly 100 billion neurons interconnected by trillions of synaptic connections in complex circuits that process vast amounts of information. Unsurprisingly, such complexity presents formidable challenges, and tools for studying brain circuits are only now being developed. Another difficulty is a lack of good model systems for brain research. Animal models used to study brain structure and function have been useful, but there are key molecular, cellular, and organizational differences between the brains of rodents or even nonhuman primates and those of humans. Perhaps for this reason, treatments for diseases that have shown promise in animal models are often ineffective in humans (Hyman, 2018; King, 2018; Sierksma et al., 2020).

Over the past few decades, neuroscientists have greatly advanced understanding of how neurons develop, function, form complex circuits, and underlie at least some simple behaviors, to the point that it is now possible to begin using this knowledge to tackle human disease mechanisms and design effective therapies. However, making this leap is difficult largely because of practical, ethical, and legal limitations to studying the human brain. Noninvasive techniques such as functional MRI (magnetic resonance imaging) or EEG (electroencephalography) provide insight into the functioning brain, but they are limited in spatial resolution, physiological information, and the types of experimental manipulations that are possible. Investigating the cellular and molecular bases of brain function requires access to brain tissue, which is difficult to obtain and generally limited

INTRODUCTION   *13*

to samples removed during surgery or postmortem. Therefore, novel methods for assessing the function and dysfunction of the human brain are needed.

To address these limitations, researchers in recent years have developed new models to better represent the human brain. The three models considered in this report are human neural organoids, human neural cell transplants (sometimes called xenografts), and human neural chimeras (see Chapter 2 for further detail).

Human neural organoids (see Figure 1-1) are three-dimensional aggregates of neural cells grown in the laboratory from human stem cells. While small (currently no more than 4 mm in diameter), neural organoids recapitulate some important developmental and molecular features of fetal human brains. Current neural organoids are limited in complexity and maturity, but researchers are working to overcome these limitations.

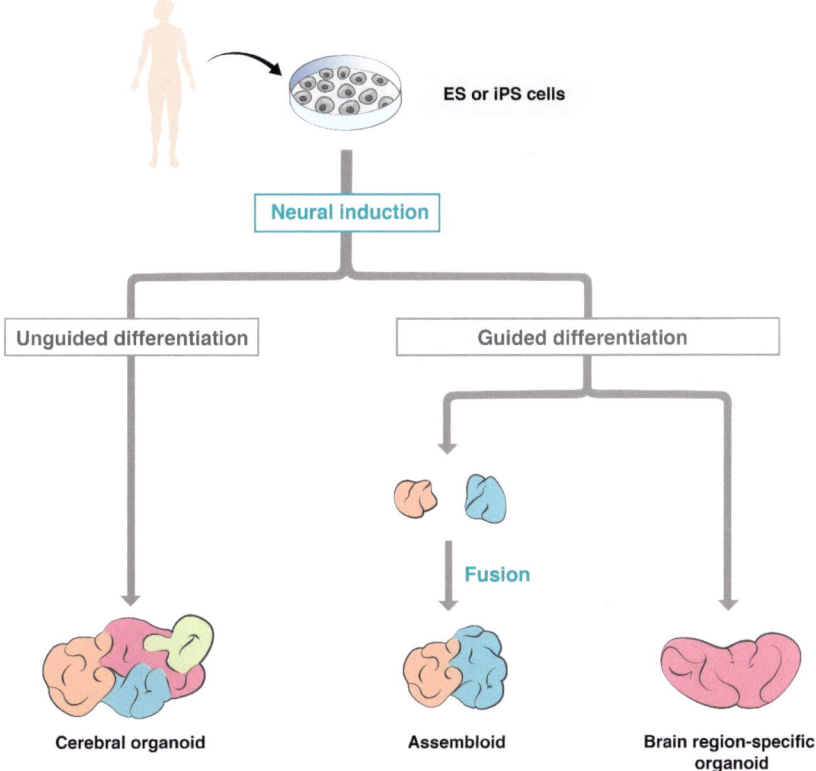

FIGURE 1-1 Human neural organoids and assembloids. Embryonic stem cells (ESCs) or induced pluripotent stem cells (iPSCs) are cultured under conditions that favor neural differentiation. In suspension, they form complex structures that share features with multiple (unguided differentiation) or single (guided differentiation) parts of the brain. Aggregates similar to distinct parts can be cultured together in close proximity to form assembloids.
IMAGE SOURCE: Maria Diaz de la Loza, Ph.D.

Human neural transplants[1] (see Figure 1-2 A, B) are generated by transplanting human cells into the brains of model organisms. Although human cells have been transplanted into nonhuman animals for decades, the range of applications has steadily increased. How extensively the human cells grow and integrate into an animal brain depends on the developmental stages of the cells and of the host brain, with earlier transplantation and less differentiated donor cells leading to more extensive codevelopment and integration. These transplants enable the study of human brain cells in the context of a whole organism and its behaviors.

Human neural chimeras (see Figure 1-2 C) are a special case of transplants. To generate a chimera, human stem cells are injected into a nonhuman host very early in embryonic development. They then intermingle with the host cells that form the brain, thereby populating it from the earliest stage and developing in parallel with the host. In one variant of the method, called blastocyst complementation, the transplanted stem cells replace many of the host cells in particular brain regions. To date, viable neural chimeras have been generated only using rodent stem cells injected into rodent hosts, but research in this area is advancing rapidly. These methods may never be applicable to humans therapeutically, but their potential as a research model is great.

While the committee focused on issues related to human neural organoids, transplants, and chimeras, such research is part of a larger field wherein analogous methods are being applied to variety of organs, such as the kidney and liver. As with neuroscience research, work in other areas has the multiple aims of elucidating developmental principles, analyzing disease mechanisms, and identifying novel therapeutic targets. For nonneural chimeras, a stated aim is to generate human organs in nonhuman hosts for potential transplantation into humans with organ failure. While the committee took note of this groundbreaking work, the current report is limited in scope to discussions of human neural organoids, transplants, and chimeras.

STUDY CHARGE

Human neural organoids, transplants, and chimeras are already yielding important insights into the functioning of the human brain and human brain disorders. As they become more like real human brains and improve as model systems, however, they raise difficult ethical questions: As human brain organoids become larger and more complex, could they gain some degree of consciousness? Could they "feel" pain? As scientists successfully integrate more human cells into the brains of chimeric animals, could the resulting animal have capacities substantially different from those typical of their species? If so, would they

---

[1] In this report, human neural transplant refers to the transplantation of human neural cells or groups of human neural cells into the brains of nonhuman animals. The transplantation of large portions of the human brain has not been proposed to date and is currently infeasible. Such transplants are excluded from consideration in this report.

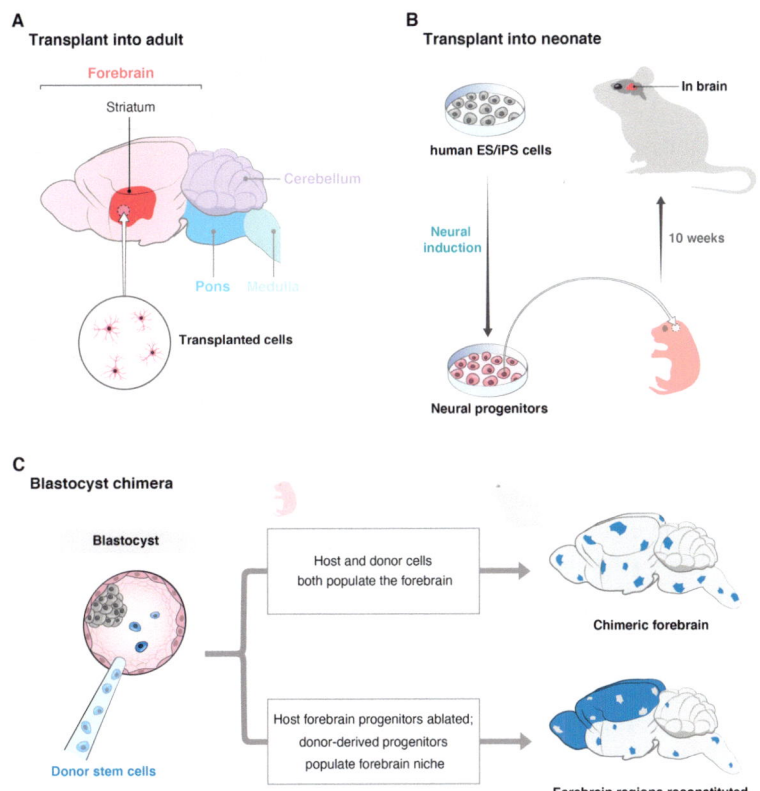

FIGURE 1-2 Human neural cell transplants and chimeras. (A) Transplantation of neural cells into specific regions of the adult brain. This sketch illustrates transplantation of cells into the striatum to replace dopaminergic neurons lost in Parkinson's disease. (B) Transplantation of neural cells into the brain of a neonatal host, whereupon they can populate multiple brain regions as the animal matures. (C) Formation of a blastocyst chimera, in which donor cells can populate the entire host brain. If host cells that form the forebrain are ablated, the host can develop with a forebrain composed largely of donor cells, a process called blastocyst complementation.
IMAGE SOURCE: Maria Diaz de la Loza, Ph.D.

need to be treated differently than other laboratory animals? Could the animals develop characteristics that are commonly thought of as human? Does creating these transplants or chimeras violate the distinction between humans and other animals that is deeply embedded in many cultures?

This report, funded by the National Institutes of Health and the Dana Foundation, examines the state of human neural organoid, transplant, and chimera research and considers some of these questions. The committee convened by the National Academies of Sciences, Engineering, and Medicine to conduct this study was asked to review the status of this research, consider its benefits and risks, examine associated ethical issues, and consider what oversight mechanisms might be appropriate in this area. In contrast to many reports produced by the National Academies, and as directed by the charge to the committee, this report provides consensus findings on these topics but not specific recommendations. The committee was asked to consider such questions as

- How would researchers define or identify enhanced or human awareness in a chimeric animal?
- Do research animals with enhanced capabilities require different treatment compared to typical animal models? What are appropriate disposal mechanisms for such models?
- What types of brain tissue are appropriate for use as neural organoids?
- How large or complex would the ex vivo brain organoids need to be to attain enhanced or human awareness?
- What kind of "humanized" brain, in size and structures, would be acceptable in a research animal?
- Should patients give explicit consent for their cells to be used to create neural organoids?
- What regulatory mechanisms relating to organoid and chimeric animal research are currently in place? Are there gaps in the current regulatory framework?
- What regulatory mechanisms exist for similar research?
- What further regulatory mechanisms might be appropriate?

Examination of these issues required both assessment of the relevant science and consideration of ethical and philosophical issues related to humanness, consciousness, self-awareness, and the welfare of entities with altered or "enhanced" capacities. To carry out these tasks, the committee conducted an extensive literature review and held seven virtual meetings in which experts provided diverse perspectives in the areas of neuroscience, animal models, theories of consciousness, religious scholarship, and other relevant areas. The committee then consolidated the information obtained to formulate the findings presented in this report as guidance for scientists, clinicians, regulators, and the general public when considering how to balance the value of this research with the ethical concerns it raises. Agendas for the committee's meetings are found in Appendix B.

ORGANIZATION OF THE REPORT

Chapter 2 summarizes the state of the science of human neural organoids, transplants, and chimeras. It also provides information on current understanding of consciousness, awareness, and related capacities, and considers how these capacities might be observed and measured in these model systems. Chapter 3 focuses on ethical issues that arise in the course of research with human neural organoids, transplants, and chimeras. Some of these issues (such as animal welfare and consent from human subjects who provide tissue for research) are the same as those encountered in other areas of biomedical research, while others are more specific to the types of research discussed in this report. Chapter 4 summarizes current oversight of research involving human neural organoids, transplants, and chimeras, which occurs at different levels—the institution where the research is taking place; professional guidelines; state and federal laws and regulations; and, for international collaborations, regulations in other countries. This chapter also considers areas in which the current oversight system might be augmented to take account of the new technologies involved in this research. Chapter 5 considers the role of public engagement in the context of emerging issues of science, technology, and medicine. The information detailed in these chapters, which was gathered through the processes described above, served as the basis for committee deliberations and for the findings presented in Chapter 6.

2

The Science of Human Neural Organoids, Transplants, and Chimeras

Neurological and psychiatric disorders take a tremendous toll (Gooch et al., 2017). Together they represent the leading cause of morbidity worldwide and account for substantial mortality. Their lifetime prevalence in the aggregate exceeds 30 percent of the population. The suffering they cause is enormous; indeed, two of the five disabilities Americans most fear are Alzheimer's disease and irreversible blindness (Scott et al., 2016), both of which result from loss of neurons. As discussed in Chapter 1, their economic impact, in the United States and globally, is massive as well in terms of both direct health care costs and indirect costs, such as lost productivity (Trautmann et al., 2016). And their incidence profile is devastating: Psychiatric diseases, which lead to lifelong disability, typically manifest by the early 20s, while lethal neurodegenerative diseases are age-related and are therefore likely to increase two-fold or more in the next few decades as the population ages.

Given the frequency and burden of brain disorders, a large community of researchers is working to understand and treat them. Progress has been slow, however, for at least three reasons. First, the brain is by far the most complex of human organs, with nearly 100 billion neurons (plus an even larger number of glial cells) comprising thousands of distinct types, interconnected in complex circuits, with some neurons making or receiving thousands of synaptic connections (see Box 2-1). Second, tools needed to probe these circuits—such as methods with which to measure activity from hundreds to thousands of neurons at the same time, to map connectivity in comprehensive ways, or to characterize the molecular differences among neuronal types or between normal and dysfunctional neurons—are still being developed. Third, while small animal and cell culture models of human disease have been extremely valuable, their limitations have been widely recognized and are particularly acute for brain disorders (Sierksma et al., 2020). Brains and brain cells of mice and rats, the most commonly used model species, differ from those of humans with respect to their size, structure, molecular composition, and pharmacological responses (Hodge et al., 2019). Furthermore, mice are most useful in modeling diseases that are caused by mutations in single genes, which can be manipulated in the mouse genome. In contrast, most prevalent human brain diseases are polygenic, meaning that their genetic underpinnings result from the combined effects of many genomic variants; at present, these complex genotypes cannot be replicated in model organisms (Hyman, 2018; Quadrato et al., 2016). Another limitation is that some neural disorders are likely due to defects in brain regions that are difficult to study in mice. For example, the prefrontal cortex, which plays a key role in executive function, is extremely underdeveloped in mice relative to humans (Wise, 2008); and the leading cause of irreversible blindness in the United States—age-related

---

BOX 2-1
The Nervous System

The nervous system is an information-processing organ of enormous complexity. It receives sensory information of many modalities, integrates and processes it, and organizes our responses. It also underlies mental activities that do not rely on immediate sensory input or lead to immediately observable behavior—for example, cognition, memory, imagination, dreaming, decision making, and self-awareness. No two people have identical nervous systems, and the variations, which result from both genetic and experiential differences among people, account for individual personalities and mental capacities. Malfunction of nervous system cells and circuits underlie all neurological and psychiatric disorders, as well as most irreversible blindness.

Parts of the nervous system (see Figure 2-1 A). The nervous system of all mammals, including humans, follows a similar general plan. The most fundamental division is into peripheral and central parts. The peripheral nervous system comprises the cells and nerves that bring sensory input to the central nervous system and relay its commands to elicit behaviors. Perhaps best known are such sensations as touch, temperature, and nociception (which elicits pain), and commands that lead to movement of muscles. These functions are mediated by the sensory and motor components of the peripheral nervous system, respectively. The peripheral nervous system also monitors and modifies a person's internal milieu—for example, sensing stomach distension and blood composition, and controlling blood pressure and heart rate. The commands to internal organs are mediated by a third peripheral division, called the autonomic nervous system.

The most fundamental division of the central nervous system is into the brain and spinal cord. The spinal cord receives inputs from the sensory division of the peripheral nervous system and sends commands to muscles and viscera through the motor and autonomic divisions. In simple cases, such as the knee-jerk reflex or withdrawal from intense heat, it mediates the entire transaction, but for more complex computations, including all conscious sensation and willed movement, it must exchange messages with the brain. The brain also receives some sensory

macular degeneration—results from loss of light-sensitive neurons in a structure called the macula that is completely absent in mice (Bringmann et al., 2018). There are also many cell types that are unique to primates or differ in gene expression between rodents and primates (see, e.g., Oberheim et al., 2009; Krienen et al., 2020). These and other differences limit the value of model organisms for research aimed at understanding the human brain, and are likely to account at least in part for the frequent failure of potential therapies developed in current animal neurological disease models to translate effectively to humans (King, 2018; Sierksma et al., 2020). The problem is more dire still for psychiatric diseases. Such disorders as autism and schizophrenia are characterized and defined by disruptions of behaviors that may not be present and certainly cannot be adequately measured in mice (Pankevich et al., 2014).

---

input directly—for example, from the eyes (visual), ears (auditory), nose (olfactory), and tongue (gustatory). It is in the brain that the most sophisticated information processing occurs. Despite the existence of individual variations, the brain's organization is extremely similar among individuals.

The brain. The brain is conventionally divided into three parts—hindbrain, midbrain, and forebrain—each with numerous subdivisions. Although it is increasingly clear that most neural functions require interactions among multiple regions, there are clear lead roles of individual regions in many mental activities. For example, distinct portions of the hindbrain control so-called vegetative functions, such as respiration and heart rate. The cerebellum, also in the hindbrain, has a key role in muscle and reflex coordination. Centers in the midbrain receive auditory and visual input and generate responses that do not reach consciousness, such as oculomotor (eye movement) reflexes and startle responses. During development, a set of cells from the forebrain grows into the eye to form the retina, which senses light, processes visual information, and passes it through the optic nerve to the rest of the brain. Structures within the forebrain include the thalamus, which relays information to the cortex, and the hypothalamus, which is the master regulator of the endocrine system, mediating unconscious drives ranging from hunger, thirst, and temperature control to sex and maternal behavior. The most rostral (anterior) part of the forebrain, which is most expanded in humans, is the telencephalon.

The telencephalon. The telenchephalon contains structures most associated with "higher functions," including the hippocampus, required for declarative memory (memory of events); the striatum, involved in decision making; and, most prominently, the cerebral cortex. Differences in cortical size among vertebrates are correlated with their cognitive capacity, both in absolute terms and relative to overall brain size. The cortex is barely present in nonmammalian vertebrates, small in rodents, larger in carnivores, larger still in nonhuman primates, and largest in humans. In primates, it can be divided into more than 100 areas by histological criteria, with functions having been assigned to many of them (see Figure 2-1 C). Some are selectively responsive to sensory stimuli of single modalities, while others, called "association areas," integrate multiple modalities.

Continued

> **BOX 2-1 Continued**
>
> The prefrontal cortex, which is, as the name implies, at the front of the cortex, is implicated in so-called executive functions, such as planning and impulse control. Association areas and prefrontal cortex occupy a larger fraction of cortical volume in humans than in other animals, and lesion studies support their involvement in higher cognitive function.
>
> *Neurons.* Most cells in the nervous system fall into one of two classes—neurons or glia (see Figure 2-2 A, C). Neurons perform most information processing. They are excitable, meaning they generate electrical signals that can be conducted within a neuron and transmitted from one neuron to another. Each neuron has a cell body, similar to that of cells throughout the body, but it differs from other cells in having long, thin processes that arise from the cell body and form connections, called synapses, with other neurons. There are two types of processes, axons and dendrites, often highly branched. Typically, electrical signals arise in dendrites and propagate through the cell body and out the axon, which forms synapses on dendrites of other neurons. At synapses, the electrical signal causes release from a presynaptic specialization of a chemical, called a neurotransmitter, which activates receptors on the abutting postsynaptic specialization. Receptor activation leads to generation of electrical signals in the postsynaptic cell or, in some cases, attenuates signals from other inputs; these are called excitatory and inhibitory synapses, respectively. The majority of neuroactive drugs, including those used to treat psychiatric illnesses (for example, antipsychotics and antidepressants) and drugs of abuse (for example, amphetamines, cocaine, and nicotine), act at synapses by increasing or inhibiting the effects of neurotransmitters.
>
> The complexity of neural function arises not only from its vast number of neurons and the complexity of their interconnections but also from neuronal variety.

Responding to the limitations of animal models, scientists have developed several ways to analyze the human brain directly. Several methods, including magnetic resonance imaging (MRI), functional MRI (fMRI), and positron emission tomography (PET), are noninvasive, allowing studies of the structure, function, and in some cases molecular composition of the human brain in awake, living individuals (Filippi, 2015). However, the spatial resolution of these methods does not allow analysis at the cellular level, and the temporal resolution is 100-fold less than that needed to capture key neural signals. Moreover, even when these modalities can detect markers of disease or disease progression, protections afforded to human subjects limit the ability to test interventions or potential therapies in human beings. Higher resolution is provided using living brain tissue removed during surgery (often for intractable epilepsy) or obtained postmortem. Slices of such ex vivo brain tissue have been used for analyses of neural activity and molecular composition of defined regions and cell types but are severely limited in quality and quantity. Moreover, when they come from patients with neurological diseases, conclusions drawn from them may not be applicable to normal subjects or to patients with other diseases. Researchers have

> There are thousands of neuronal types, which differ in numerous characteristics, including their size, their shape, the branching patterns of their axons and dendrites, and their electrical properties. They also use many chemical signals, including some 10 neurotransmitters, which mediate synaptic interactions on a millisecond time scale, as well as dozens of neuromodulatory agents, which affect synaptic signaling on slower time scales. Each region of the brain may contain 100 or more cell types, with highly specific connections among them. Many connections are specified genetically during embryonic development, but a main way in which experience shapes the nervous system is by remodeling patterns of connectivity in postnatal life.
>
> *Glia.* Although neurons get most of the attention, they are actually outnumbered by glial cells. Once thought to provide primarily mechanical support (the term glia comes from the Greek word for glue), they are now known to provide many supporting functions, and also to participate in signaling. The three glial classes of the central nervous system are astrocytes, oligodendrocytes, and microglia (see Figure 2-2 C). Astrocytes promote synapse formation and function; oligodendrocytes form myelin that acts as insulating material around axons, speeding conduction of electrical signals; and microglia are surveillance cells that respond to injuries and insults, both removing debris and regulating inflammation. Loss of oligodendrocytes leads to so-called demyelinating diseases, the most prominent of which is multiple sclerosis. Astrocytes and microglia have recently been implicated in the pathogenesis of many brain disorders, including autism and Alzheimer's disease. In the peripheral nervous system, a single glial type, the Schwann cell, carries out roles of all three central glial types.

also generated cultures from human neurons or stem cells induced to form neurons (discussed further below), but these two-dimensional cultures fail to form stereotyped, complex circuits.

Experimental models of the human brain are therefore needed. As discussed in Chapter 1, three sets of model systems have been developed that allow scientists to analyze human neural cells in powerful new ways: neural organoids, neural cell transplants, and neural chimeras. In this report we refer to these three systems according to the following definitions:

- *Neural organoids* are three-dimensional cultures derived from pluripotent stem cells that have been treated in ways that lead them to generate neurons and glia (see Figure 1-1 in Chapter 1). Organoids can contain multiple neuronal and glial cell types and, unlike classical neuronal cultures, exhibit complex synaptic interactions among types. They represent an important complement to conventional "monolayer" cell cultures and animal models.
- *Neural cell transplants.* Neural cells or, in some cases, neural organoids, can be transplanted directly into the brain of a nonhuman animal, either

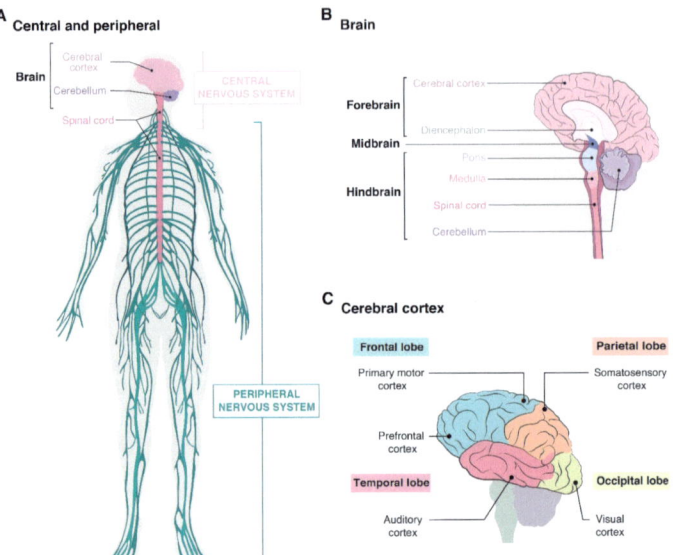

FIGURE 2-1 Architecture of the human nervous system. (A) Motor, sensory, and autonomic nerves of the peripheral nervous system connect the central nervous system to the body. The figure shows nerve trunks of the peripheral nervous system but not its numerous ganglia, most of which lie adjacent to the spinal cord. The central nervous system is composed of the brain and spinal cord. (B) The three major subdivisions of the brain are forebrain, midbrain, and hindbrain, each of which is subdivided into multiple regions, each with primary responsibility for distinct sets of functions. (C) Cerebral cortex, showing the four lobes, as well as several key areas with known functions.
IMAGE SOURCE: Maria Diaz de la Loza, Ph.D.

during development or in adulthood. They are examples of "xenotransplants," a term that refers to insertion of cells from one species into a host of another species. Transplanted neuronal precursors can mature into functional neurons and integrate into the host nervous system, receiving synaptic inputs from and providing synaptic input to host neurons. Transplanted glia can also interact with host cells. Cells in neural cell transplants vary in where and how they interact with the recipient's brain, but they seldom if ever contribute to other host tissues or organs.

- *Neural chimeras* are a form of transplant in which donor cells are introduced into the nonhuman animal at an embryonic stage prior to formation of the nervous system. The donor cells can therefore develop in parallel with host cells, enabling high levels of integration. In some cases, host cells of particular types are ablated by genetic methods, so donor cells injected at a very early stage (the blastocyst) can provide the major contribution to a tissue or organ. This method is called blastocyst complementation.

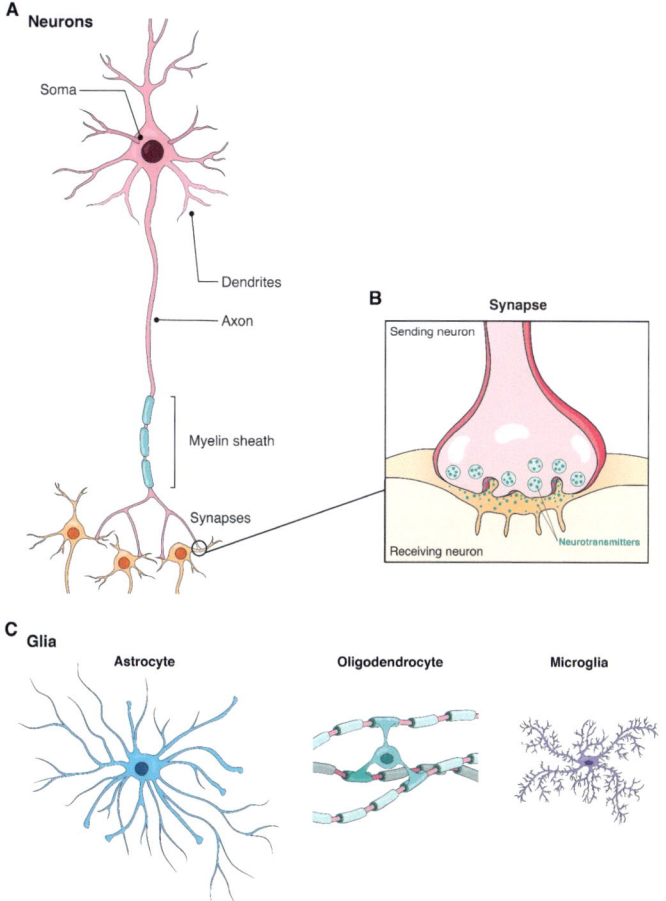

FIGURE 2-2 Cells of the nervous system. (A) A neuron, showing multiple dendrites and a single axon extending from the cell body (soma). Information generally flows in through dendrites and out through axons. Axons of one neuron form synapses on dendrites of other neurons. (B) A synapse. Electrical signals in axons lead to release of neurotransmitter released from a nerve terminal; the transmitter then activates receptors on the postsynaptic cell to generate new signals. (C) Major glial types: astrocyte, oligodendrocyte, and microglia.
IMAGE SOURCE: Maria Diaz de la Loza, Ph.D.

The distinction between a neural cell transplant and a neural chimera rests largely on whether the introduced cells remain limited to the nervous system or contribute substantially to other organs. This distinction is not always clear-cut in practice. A useful dividing line at present is the gastrula stage of embryogenesis, at which cells are fated to generate specific organs. In general, scientists in the field view introduction of exogenous cells to an organism prior to gastrulation as generating chimeras and after gastrulation as generating transplants.

Organoids and in vivo animal models that are derived from or incorporate human neural cells have raised ethical and philosophical concerns, based in part on the use of human material and in part on the capabilities they might acquire. As the methods become more powerful, these concerns will intensify. The remainder of this chapter surveys the current state of these technologies and considers likely improvements over the next several years. Because many concerns about these models arise from issues related to consciousness, awareness, or sentience, the discussion includes a review of current understanding of those capacities and methods for assessing or monitoring them. Ethical and moral issues are discussed in Chapter 3, and regulatory and oversight mechanisms in Chapter 4.

HUMAN NEURAL ORGANOIDS

Organoids are three-dimensional cell cultures in which multiple cell types are arranged in patterns that recapitulate some features of the corresponding organ in vivo. They are usually derived from stem cells that have the potential to mature into many types of cells, such as embryonic stem cells (ESCs) or induced pluripotent stem cells (iPSCs) (see Figure 2-3). ESCs are obtained from early embryos, at a time when cells are still totipotent—that is, capable of differentiating into any cell type. They are maintained in culture using methods that allow them to retain this capacity. When rodent ESCs are injected into the blastocyst of the same species, they can give rise to a complete embryo. iPSCs are obtained from postnatal specimens, usually skin or blood. Cells are treated with a cocktail of factors that lead them to differentiate into a pluripotent state. They can then be used as an alternative to ESCs (see Takahashi and Yamanaka, 2006). To generate organoids, ESCs or iPSCs are cultured under conditions that promote their aggregation, growth, and differentiation into multiple cell types and the "self-assembly" of these types into structures that display features of an organ. Expanding on early attempts to generate more complex cultures (see, e.g., Zhang et al., 2001; Watanabe et al., 2007), Eiraku and colleagues (2008) used the method to generate aggregates with features characteristic of forebrain structures. This strategy was soon applied to generate organoids resembling many other tissues (Clevers, 2016; Eiraku et al., 2011; Sato et al., 2009).

Neural organoids, in which cells are predominantly if not entirely neural (i.e., neuronal or glial), are typically classified into two main groups (see Figure 1-1). In one, called self-patterning or whole-brain organoids, cells take on identities typical of multiple brain regions. They have the advantage that interactions normally occurring among regions can in principle be analyzed in a single structure. On the other hand, their organization differs vastly from that of any particular part of an actual brain, and they display high levels of organoid-to-organoid variability. In the other group, called prepatterned organoids, cells are directed to generate cells typical of specific, restricted brain regions. This class of organoid was pioneered by Sasai and colleagues, who showed that supplementing the

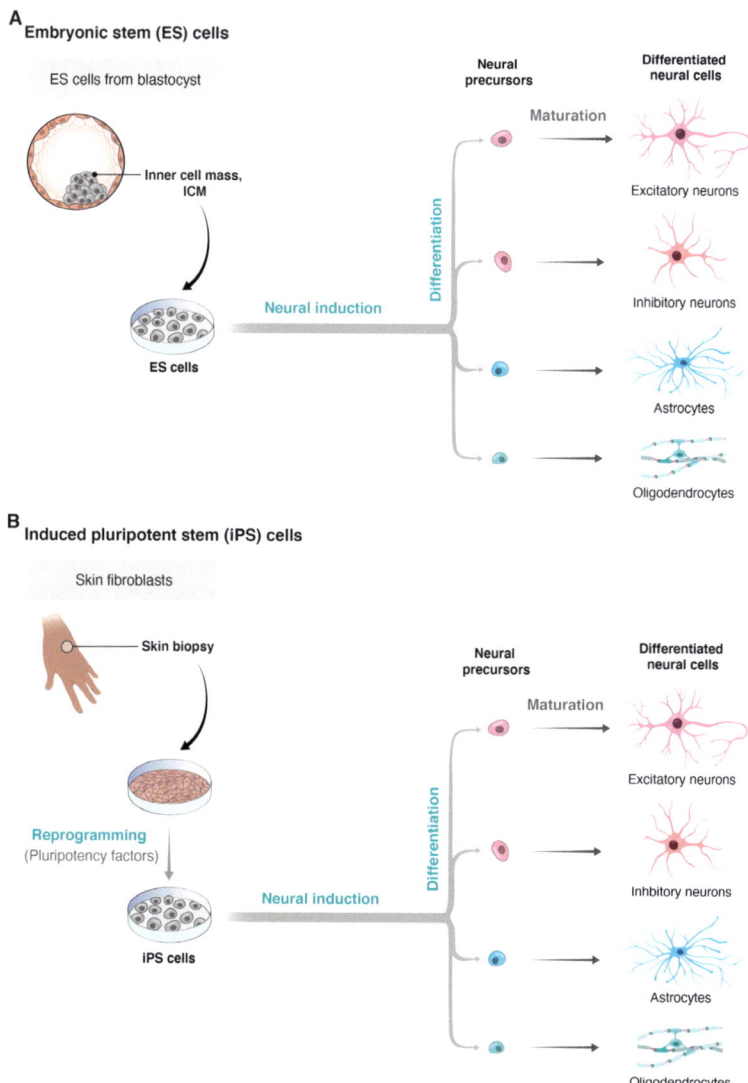

FIGURE 2-3 Embryonic stem cells (ESCs) and induced pluripotent stem cells (iPSCs). ESCs and iPSCs can be treated to differentiate into a variety of neural cell types. (A) ESCs are generated from cells of the inner cell mass of blastocysts. (B) iPSCs are generated from adult skin fibroblasts. Both ESCs and iPSCs can be maintained and expanded in culture, and treated to differentiate into neural progenitor cells. The progenitors can be induced to differentiate into specific neural cell types in monolayer cultures or organoids (see Figure 1-1) or transplanted into host animals (see Figure 1-2 A, B). Undifferentiated ESCs or iPSCs can also be injected into a blastocyst to generate a chimera (see Figure 1-2 C).
IMAGE SOURCE: Maria Diaz de la Loza, Ph.D.

media with agents known to regulate neural development in vivo and including extracellular matrix components (for better scaffolding) (Ueno, et al., 2006) could influence the identity of the structures that formed—for example, causing them to resemble distinct parts of the forebrain. Later, protocols were developed to generate organoids with some characteristics of other regions, including striatum, retina, thalamus, and spinal cord (Andersen et al., 2020; Cowan et al., 2020; Kadoshima et al., 2013; Miura et al., 2020; Velasco et al., 2019).

For self-organizing cortical organoids, pioneering work was reported by Lancaster and colleagues (2013), who devised standardized methods for generating organoids from iPSCs and demonstrated the self-organizing capacity of whole-brain organoids. Building on this work, many groups have improved the method to extend culture times (to more than 9 months) and to recapitulate key features of brain development, such as neurogenesis from progenitor zones, patterns of gene activity, migration of specific cell types, aspects of neural circuitry, and generation of spontaneous and induced electrical activity (Le Bail et al., 2020; Pasca, 2018; Quadrato et al., 2017). Using patient-derived iPSCs and stem cells engineered to carry mutations associated with human diseases, organoids have provided insight into several human diseases (see Figure 2-4).

For example, Lancaster and colleagues (2013) generated iPSCs from a patient with microcephaly caused by a mutation in a specific gene (CDK5RAP2) and showed that neural organoids derived from that cell line exhibited features characteristic of the disease. Subsequently, researchers used neural organoids to investigate neurodevelopmental changes in individuals with severe idiopathic autism spectrum disorder, elucidating molecular mechanisms that underlie overproduction of inhibitory neurons (Mariani et al., 2015). Cells from individuals with 22q11.2 deletion syndrome (DiGeorge syndrome) were differentiated into neural organoids to identify defects in spontaneous neuronal activity and calcium signaling commonly associated with this syndrome and other genetic forms of the neuropsychiatric disease (Khan et al., 2018). Ye and colleagues (2017) produced organoids from cells donated by a schizophrenia patient with a mutation in a gene called DISC1 (disrupted-in-schizophrenia 1) and documented significant disruptions in cellular processes caused by the mutation. Birey and colleagues (2017) analyzed Timothy syndrome, a devastating neurodevelopmental disorder, in a similar way. Neural organoids have also been valuable in investigating the mechanisms underlying Zika virus (ZIKV)–associated microcephaly in infants, with ZIKV-infected human iPSC-derived neural organoids showing a range of neurodevelopmental abnormalities (Birey et al., 2017; Qian et al., 2017). More recently, these models were used to elucidate the effects of SARS-CoV-2 on the choroid plexus and the blood–brain barrier (Pellegrini et al., 2020).

Organoids differ from the human brain in several significant respects. First, they are small, generally less than 4 mm in diameter, and contain fewer than 2–3 million cells. In contrast, an adult human brain measures approximately 1,350 cubic centimeters and contains some 100 billion cells (neurons and glia)—an

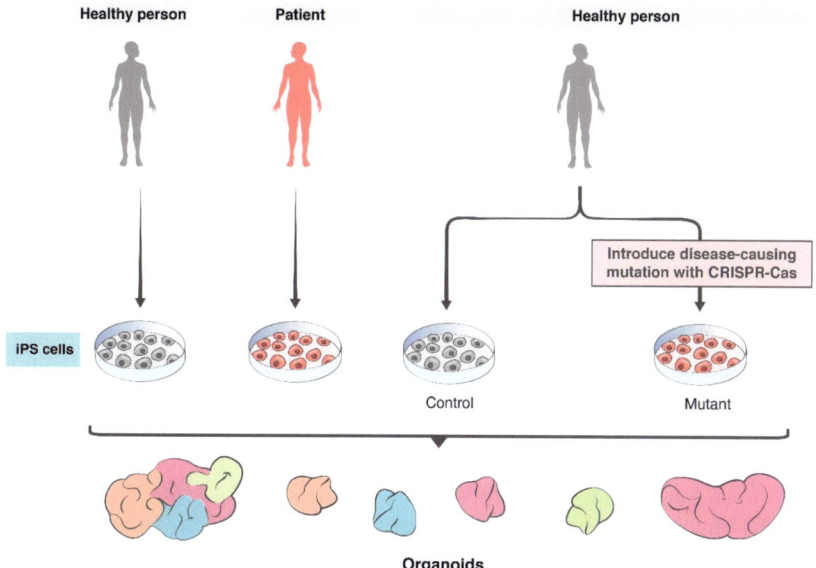

FIGURE 2-4 Use of induced pluripotent stem cells (iPSCs) to analyze mechanisms of brain disease. Organoids derived from patients with specific brain disorders can be used to analyze mechanisms underlying the disorder. In one strategy (left), organoids are generated from iPSCs obtained from healthy donors and patients. The organoids are then compared to seek abnormalities in structure, function, or molecular composition that correlate with and possibly account for some disease phenotypes. In another strategy, iPSCs obtained from a healthy donor are subjected to genome editing to introduce mutations or variants that have been associated with a particular disease. Organoids are then generated from the edited and unedited cells and compared. In both strategies, organoids that exhibit abnormalities associated with a disease can be used to screen compounds that might form the basis for therapeutic approaches.
IMAGE SOURCE: Maria Diaz de la Loza, Ph.D.

approximately 40,000-fold difference. One major constraint on growth is that neural organoids do not have blood vessels to supply oxygen and nutrients or to remove metabolic waste, so their size is limited in part by diffusion. Moreover, the hypoxic (oxygen-poor) core can become necrotic. Second, organoids do not recapitulate characteristics of many brain regions, and therefore cannot form the complex networks of connections among regions that typify the brain. Third, at present, circuits that do form lack many features that underlie information processing in the brain. For example, while major cell classes are represented, neural organoids do not display the full diversity of individual cell types found in the brain, nor do they exhibit patterns of organization, lamination, and precise connectivity observed in vivo (Bhaduri et al., 2020; Velasco et al., 2020). Fourth, most neural organoids lack cells of nonneural origin, such as microglia, endothelial cells, and vascular cells, that are critical for brain health and function. Finally, the neurons, glia, and synapses that form in organoids currently fail to mature beyond those stages typically found in neonatal brains, limiting their utility for analyzing the mature human brain.

Researchers are working to overcome these limitations (Del Dosso et al., 2020). Recent and ongoing efforts include the following:

- *Vascularization.* Providing organoids with a blood supply would, in principle, give the interior of the organoid access to oxygen and nutrients and enable the elimination of waste products. It is unclear, however, whether vascularization alone would enable growth to a larger size. Vessels are generated from nonneural cells, so they are not present in organoids formed from neural stem cells. Researchers are working to integrate synthetic vasculature into the three-dimensional matrix used for organoid formation (Karzbrun and Reiner, 2019). Alternatively, when neural organoids are implanted into the brains of adult mice, host vessels invade the implant and supply it with nutrients (Mansour et al., 2018). In this case, the organoid and host brain can also become synaptically interconnected.
- *Long-range connectivity among brain regions.* Connections among multiple brain regions are required for most neural computations in the nervous system and all motor behaviors and perceptions. Currently, many organoids contain a mixture of cells that resemble those found in multiple regions, but without the cellular organization or regional segregation found in the brain. In other cases, organoids are generated under conditions that favor differentiation into structures resembling a single region, such as the cerebral cortex or the retina. In neither case can orderly long-range connections form. As a way to promote orderly and predictable long-range connectivity, an "assembloid" method has been devised in which organoids are grown separately under conditions that promote their acquisition of features characteristic of distinct regions (see Figure 1-1). They are then placed in close proximity to each other, whereupon they form interregional connections (Birey et al., 2017). The most recent studies include combinations of organoids directed to differentiate into aggregates resembling cortex, striatum, spinal cord, and skeletal muscle (Andersen et al., 2020; Miura et al., 2020).
- *Individual variation among organoids.* Variation among organoids was a vexing problem in early studies, even for organoids generated from the same iPSC line and cultured under seemingly identical conditions. This variability impeded the ability to identify, for example, disease- or patient-specific features. More recently, standardization of conditions has led to a decrease in this variability (Cowan et al., 2020; Velasco et al., 2019; Yoon et al., 2019).
- *Use of microfluidic devices (Rifes et al., 2020; Uzel et al., 2016) and specialized materials (Sood et al., 2019).* Use of these methods to sup-

port organoid formation enables greater control over the size, uniformity, and patterning of the organoids. As these methods improve, they may also help address issues of reproducibility and generation of higher-order structure.

The major unaddressed limitation is immaturity. Neither neurons nor glia mature to typical adult states in organoids generated to date (Bhaduri et al., 2020). Several groups are using innovative methods to enhance neuronal survival and axon outgrowth and to maintain organoids for longer periods (Giandomenico et al., 2019, 2020), but the inability to model adult patterns of gene expression or connectivity in organoids is a persistent problem. Nonetheless, recent and foreseeable advances hold promise that the use of organoids can advance from modeling disease to providing a platform for testing potential treatments. Already, Esk and colleagues (2020) have been able to screen organoids to identify genes responsible for microcephaly; based on the results of the screen, they elucidated a dysregulated intracellular signaling pathway that led to the disease phenotype. Nonneural organoids are already being used for drug screens (Driehuis et al. 2019; Schuster et al., 2020), with parallel efforts using neural organoids in progress. The future will surely see increased use of iPSCs obtained from adults for whom extensive phenotypic and genotypic data are available; from people with complex polygenic diseases; from children with diseases that are fatal before adulthood; and from patients with diseases in which nonneural symptoms complicate analysis of neurological features. These patient-specific organoids present a unique opportunity for modeling diseases and testing potential treatments (see Figure 2-4).

HUMAN NEURAL TRANSPLANTS

There is a long history of transplanting neural progenitors from one animal into the brain of another. Among the first such efforts were studies aimed at treating Parkinson's disease. Parkinson's results from the death of dopaminergic neurons, so several groups proposed implanting dopaminergic precursors or progenitors derived from fetal tissue into patients with the disease to replace those that had been lost (see Figure 1-2 A). Studies in rodent and then nonhuman primate models in the 1970s led to initial clinical trials in patients in the 1980s (Sladek and Gash, 1988). Although efficacy was insufficient for expanded use, results were sufficiently encouraging that efforts in this line of research continue to this day (Kim et al., 2020). This pioneering work also paved the way for many groups to transplant neuronal progenitors derived from rodent embryos or rodent neuronal cell lines into multiple sites within the neonatal rodent brain, with the dual aims of studying neuronal development and testing therapeutic potential (see Figure 1-2 B) (Björklund and Lindvall, 2000).

A major advance came with the ability to generate neurons from human stem cells, particularly iPSCs. As was the case for organoids, discussed above, these reagents freed the field from reliance on scarce and ethically challenging fetal tissue. In appropriate mouse models, for example, transplantation of midbrain neuronal progenitors generated from human embryonic stem cells attenuates Parkinsonian symptoms (Kim et al., 2020; Xiong et al., 2020); transplantation of interneurons generated from iPSCs attenuates epilepsy (Cunningham et al., 2014; Harward and Southwell, 2020; Southwell et al., 2014; Upadhya et al., 2019); and transplantation of similar inhibitory interneurons into spinal cord attenuates neuropathic pain (Braz et al., 2017; Hunt and Baraban, 2015). Other studies have transplanted small numbers of neurons derived from human iPSCs into mouse cortex and studied them with histological and physiological methods to analyze human-specific developmental features that would not be accessible using human fetal material (Linaro et al., 2019). In addition, to investigate disease mechanisms, stem cells to be transplanted can be genetically modified or derived from patients with specific diseases (see Figure 2-4).

Finally, although the majority of transplantation studies have focused on engraftment of neuronal progenitors, exciting results have also been reported for glial transplants, including all of the three major glial types: oligodendrocytes, which form myelin; astrocytes, which support neuronal metabolism and signaling; and microglia, which are critical for responses to injury and inflammation (see Box 2-1). For example, human glial progenitors can restore oligodendrocytes that form myelin in a mutant mouse that lacks oligodendrocytes (Windrem et al., 2020). Given that several human diseases, including multiple sclerosis, result from myelin loss, this preclinical study suggests a promising therapeutic approach. In another experiment, Hasselmann and colleagues (2019) populated the mouse brain with microglia derived from human iPSCs and showed that these microglia respond to brain injury and inflammation in ways similar to endogenous microglia. Han and colleagues (2013) transplanted human astrocyte precursors into neonatal mouse cortex and found, remarkably, that as adults, the hosts exhibited improved performance in learning and memory tasks compared with controls. One possible explanation is that the human astrocytes were better able than their mouse counterparts to support the neuronal functions responsible for the behaviors.

HUMAN NEURAL CHIMERAS

Transplants vary markedly in the number and type of human neural cells introduced and the stage at which they are introduced into the nonhuman host. In general, the extent of integration is likely to be greater the earlier the cells are engrafted because they can then develop and interact in parallel with host cells. In this respect, introduction into the embryonic blastocyst of a nonhuman mammal allows maximal engraftment.

The blastocyst is a hollow ball of cells within which a small group, called the inner cell mass, is destined to give rise to the entire embryo. (The cells that form the ball itself are the precursors of the placenta.) In this method, ESCs or iPSCs are microinjected into the blastocyst cavity, where they mix with cells of the host inner cell mass (see Figure 1-2 C). The embryo is then implanted into the uterus of a female of that animal species, where it can develop to term and give rise to live, healthy, chimeric offspring. The method was initially developed for generation of genetically engineered mouse "knock-out" lines, in which genetically engineered embryonic stem cells contribute to all tissues, including the gonads, generating what are called germline chimeras. In blastocyst complementation, the host blastocyst is engineered so that cells of a particular organ either fail to form or are eliminated at an early stage. The introduced cells can still populate all tissues, but they make their greatest contribution to the eliminated organ because they do not need to compete there with host cells. Specificity can be enhanced by engineering the donor embryonic stem cells or iPSCs to eliminate their ability to generate particular cell types, most importantly germ cells. This method has been used to generate chimeric mice, rats, and pigs with donor-derived organs including pancreas, but the only chimeras generated from human cells to date have not survived past extremely early embryonic stages (Masaki and Nakauchi, 2017; Wu et al., 2017).

Recently, Chang and colleagues (2018) used blastocyst complementation to generate mice in which most forebrain neurons were derived from another mouse. They showed extensive replacement of principal (excitatory) neurons of the host by those from the mouse donor, and demonstrated that the offspring were healthy and, to the extent tested, structurally and behaviorally intact. They also generated chimeras using embryonic stem cells from a mouse in which they had inactivated a gene implicated in human intellectual disability. The offspring recapitulated structural and behavioral phenotypes characteristic of the mouse mutant, demonstrating the power of this method to model diseases.

In most chimeras described to date, the donor and host are from the same species, but in a few cases, they differ—for example, rat embryonic stem cells can contribute extensively to nonneural mouse organs (Kobayashi et al., 2010; Wu et al., 2017). At present, formation of neural chimeras from injection of human ESCs or iPSCs into mouse blastocysts has not been reported, and there are good reasons to believe it would be infeasible for brains at this time. One major impediment is that maturation times of human and mouse neurons are roughly proportional to the gestation times of the species, which differ by more than 10-fold, and the temporal mismatch persists when human neural cells are transplanted into mouse brain (Linaro et al., 2019; Masaki and Nakauchi, 2017; Rayon et al., 2020). Thus, even though the introduced human cells might begin to develop in parallel with the host mouse cells, the temporal mismatch would likely prevent formation of a functional chimeric brain. Attempts to improve integration of human cells into rodents in chimerism are under way, but the contributions to the nervous system have to date been minimal (Hu et al., 2020). It is possible that transplantation of human stem cells into a nonhuman primate with greater genetic similarity to humans and a more similar gestation time (gestation time for macaques is around 5 months) might reduce this mismatch and allow some degree of chimerism to occur. Moreover, chimeras generated in nonhuman primates may well be better models of human disorders, particularly psychiatric disorders, relative to chimeras generated in rodents. Results from macaque models of autism, generated by gene editing, support this idea (Qiu et al., 2019; Zhou et al., 2019).

CAPACITIES OF HUMAN NEURAL ORGANOIDS, TRANSPLANTS, AND CHIMERAS

Human neural organoids, transplants, and chimeras all contain neurons that can generate and propagate electrical signals (action potentials) and form synapses with other neurons. For organoids, synaptic partners are within the organoid, whereas donor neurons in transplants and chimeras can form synapses with host neurons. Neurons in organoids have already been shown to generate electrical signals in response to a sensory stimulus (light) and to evoke contractions in cocultured muscle cells (Andersen et al., 2020; Quadrato et al., 2017). Even simple neural circuits, such as those that form in conventional monolayer (two-dimensional) cultures, are capable of rudimentary information processing (Ju et al., 2015), and the same is true of neural organoids. For neural transplants and chimeras, synaptic connections with the host imply that the introduced neurons could respond to sensory inputs, influence motor outputs, and participate in sophisticated computations.

As discussed in Chapter 3, some ethical concerns about human neural organoids, transplants, and chimeras require further scientific knowledge to address, and some do not. Of those ethical concerns that require more research, the most prominent regarding neural organoids revolve around the possibility that they might develop certain capacities, such as perception, consciousness, or the ability to experience pain. These capacities are not thought to be present in current neural organoids or in monolayer culture systems. For neural transplants and chimeras, a key concern is that as a consequence of introducing human neurons, existing capacities of the host might be altered in ways that would make their experience of the world much more similar to that of humans. This concern would be heightened if the host were a nonhuman primate, because more deference is accorded to primates used in research than to other species, such as mice and rats (see below). Capacities of greatest concern include the capacity to experience pain and the quality termed consciousness.

Pain

The subjective experience of feeling pain is certainly not a uniquely human quality, and behavioral and physiological metrics for assessing pain in nonhuman animals are well established. Such measurements can be applied to animals with neural cell transplants and to chimeras. The idea that organoids now or in the future might feel pain is a more challenging and perhaps more concerning question to some.

But what is pain? At the simplest level it involves activation of a set of sensory neurons called nociceptors, which respond to such potentially damaging stimuli as corrosive chemicals, intense pressure, or extreme heat. However, pain is an experience, not simply a sensation, and nociceptors are neither necessary nor sufficient to evoke it.[1] For example, patients who have had limbs amputated sometimes report pain in those limbs even in the absence of nociceptors. Conversely, stimulation of nociceptors fails to evoke pain in the presence of analgesics that act on the central nervous system. Instead, pain may be more closely associated with activity in regions of the brain to which nociceptors project, directly or indirectly—for example, the anterior cingulate and insular regions of the cerebral cortex. Indeed, pain can be elicited by direct activation of these and other brain areas, without nociceptive stimulation (Harriott et al., 2021; Sun et al., 2020). However, these circuits remain incompletely defined, so it is difficult to provide guidance on what circuits would need to be present in an organoid for it to generate a percept akin to pain. Whatever the relevant circuits are, they are vastly more sophisticated than any circuitry present in current organoids or assembloids, and the prospects for generating such complex circuits in the foreseeable future are remote.

Even less well defined is the potential to experience pain. Some experts point to this capacity as being as important as pain itself because it does not rely on any specific stimulation paradigm. At present, however, the capacity to experience pain can be assessed only in the context of a painful stimulus. This situation may change as the circuitry required to experience pain becomes better understood, but at present neuroscientists would not be able to recognize neural circuits that confer the potential for pain in an organoid even if they existed.

Thus, two related but logically distinct concerns about pain in human neural transplants, chimeras, and organoids might be raised: that the entity actually experiences pain, and that the entity has the capacity to experience pain (or the potential to develop that capacity). Chapter 3 considers the issue of the experience of pain in research animals from the perspective of animal welfare regulations, which form the current basis for oversight of animal research, as well as from the perspective of animal rights.

Consciousness

A key capacity of concern is consciousness, sometimes termed sentience or awareness. These terms are notoriously difficult to define and are even more

---

[1] Allan Basbaum, University of California-San Francisco, presentation to the committee, August 11, 2020, virtual meeting.

difficult to measure. Because these terms are often used interchangeably, we use "consciousness" hereafter, even though its equivalence with other terms is not universally accepted.

Consciousness, in the sense that elicits substantial ethical concern, denotes a subjective experience, people's introspective awareness of the external world and the internal states of their own bodies, generally tied to a cognitive and/or emotional impact. In the absence of subjective experience, moral or ethical concerns are substantially diminished. For example, before surgery is performed on human patients (and most nonhuman animals), subjective experience is abolished by means of anesthetic drugs to prevent the experience of suffering. Entities that lack the capacity for subjective experience, such as plants, are accorded lower moral status relative to animals known or believed to have the capacity for consciousness.

A reasonable intuition for consciousness thus defined is provided by the experience of visual perception. A person's typical perception of a visual scene consists of recognizable objects and living beings that move (or do not) in familiar ways. This conscious experience is merely the tip of an iceberg of neural processing; it lies atop a vast complex of unconscious visual processing. People are not consciously aware, for example, that their brain actually receives two visual images—one from each eye—and combines them to form a conscious perception of a single world. Nor are people aware of the processing that causes them to perceive a single, stable visual world even though their eyes move a few times per second (saccades), sending changing views to the brain that must be stitched into a single perceived world. Analogous conscious experiences (and underlying icebergs of unconscious processing) exist in all sensory domains, as well as in the internal cognitive realms of learning, memory, affect, and attention.

The adoption of a working definition of consciousness is necessary for specifying ethical issues involved in research with human neural organoids, transplants, and chimeric animals. Once specified, ethical judgments could be critically informed by knowledge of underlying neural mechanisms. Many theories and definitions of consciousness are framed in ways that cannot readily be applied to brain function. In some cases, however, philosophers and neuroscientists working together have endeavored to provide explanations of consciousness that are amenable to scientific inquiry (Doerig et al., 2020; Linkenhoker, 2019). Two of the most prominent are the integrated information theory and the global workspace theory. According to the integrated information theory, consciousness is correlated with the ability of a system to integrate information (Tononi et al., 2016). Therefore, the level of consciousness in a brain could theoretically be measured and compared between species, individuals, and circumstances. The perturbational complexity index (PCI), described below, provides one potential metric. The global workspace theory holds that consciousness relates to an ongoing, changing broadcast of a person's mental contents (the tips of the unconscious processing icebergs) to a diverse network of brain circuits by means of long-range anatomical connections (Dehaene, 2014; Mashour et al., 2020).

Whatever the definition of consciousness, a key question is the extent to which it is a particularly human attribute. Higher levels of subjective experience are almost always studied in human subjects, who are able to report their experiences verbally. That does not mean, however, that consciousness is confined to humans. Indeed, the view that consciousness, particularly self-consciousness, is a defining attribute of humans has been challenged by philosophers, ethicists, animal behaviorists, and ethologists. The current consensus is that all vertebrates and some cephalopods possess consciousness to some extent. It has been suggested that mammals have a higher level of consciousness compared with non-mammalian vertebrates, primates compared with other mammals, and humans compared with other primates (DeGrazia, 2009). Few people who have lived or worked closely with vertebrate animals—for example, pet owners and research scientists—harbor any doubt that these animals have subjective experiences of the sensory world and the inner world of memory, affect, and self-movement toward goals (i.e., purpose).

Whether any of the higher levels of consciousness, such as self-awareness—that is, the ability to reflect on one's own subjective experiences—are restricted to humans remains an open question. One framework for thinking about self-awareness was proposed by DeGrazia (2009). Although his model is not explicitly framed in evolutionary terms, it maps onto phylogenetic distinctions. DeGrazia posits four levels of self-consciousness. The first, agential, is awareness that one's body is distinct from the rest of the environment and subject to one's direct control. DeGrazia argues that many vertebrates have this capacity. The second level, social, involves awareness of one's position within social relationships, such as dominance hierarchies and kinship groups. It appears to be characteristic of many mammals. The third, introspective, denotes awareness of one's own mental status, beliefs, or feelings (metacognition). Current evidence suggests that this level is well developed in primates and may be present to some degree in other mammals as well. The fourth level, autobiographical identity, involves awareness of oneself as an individual, having a rich remembered past; entertaining multiple possibilities for the future; and possessing a narrative of some sort connecting past, present, and future. This level may be specific to humans, although it may be present to some extent in their closest relatives, the great apes (e.g., chimpanzees and gorillas). This evolutionary conception of consciousness views it as a graded quality rather than one divided into distinct groups of "have" and "have not" species based on specific abilities, such as the ability of an animal to recognize itself in a mirror (the so-called "mirror self-recognition" test (see Figure 2-5) (Anderson and Gallup, 2015).

A second set of critical questions about consciousness is neurobiological: What neural circuits are required for consciousness, and where in the brain are they housed? Answers to these questions can ground judgments about the pos-

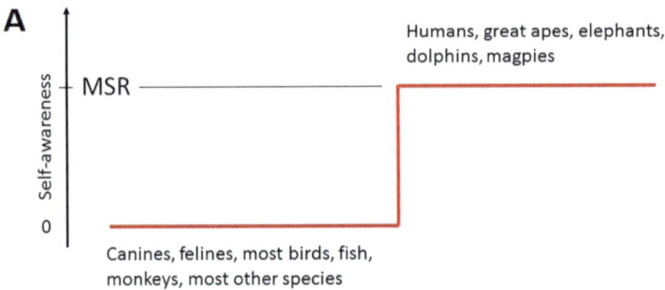

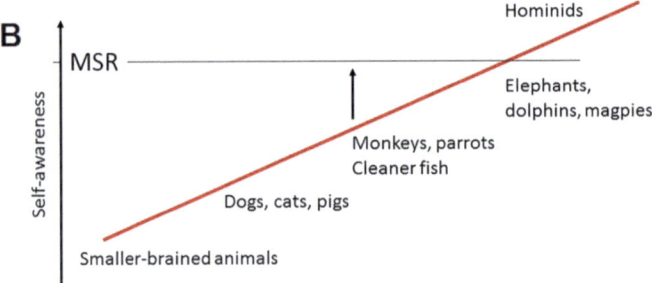

FIGURE 2-5 Distinct evolutionary views of consciousness. In the traditional binary model (A), species showing mirror self-recognition (MSR) possess a self-concept, whereas all other species do not. The gradualist view (B), in contrast, assigns the highest level of self-awareness to hominids, who spontaneously explore and play with their reflection and care about their appearance, and assigns intermediate or lower levels to other species. Reactions to mirrors range from permanent confusion about one's reflection to a certain level of understanding of how mirrors operate (e.g., using them as tools) and only brief or no confusion between one's reflection and a stranger. Some species, such as macaques and perhaps cleaner fish, appear to possess this intermediate level and can therefore, with the aid of training and/or multimodal stimulation, be "lifted" (arrow) to a level of mirror understanding closer to MSR.
SOURCE: de Waal, 2019. Copyright: © 2019 Frans B. M. de Waal. This figure is reproduced from an open access article distributed under the terms of the Creative Commons Attribution License (see https://creativecommons.org/licenses/by/4.0/), which permits unrestricted use, distribution, and reproduction in any medium, provided the original author and source are credited. The figure caption has been adapted from the original figure text.

sibilities of conscious experience in human neural organoids, transplants, and chimeras.

Research in this area has proceeded on two fronts. The first involves an attempt to define the neural circuits responsible for consciousness, often called "neural correlates of consciousness" (Koch et al., 2016). Several promising candidates have been proposed, but there is no consensus on which are most relevant. Detailed analysis of circuitry is generally carried out in model systems but has been extended to human subjects using fMRI (Dehaene, 2014; Huang et al., 2020). For example, Dehaene (2014) presents subliminal stimuli to subjects and asks which brain regions are activated by those that make the subject consciously aware of a stimulus that would otherwise not reach consciousness.

The other front for neurobiological research involves determining which brain regions house the highest levels of consciousness. Since these are, as far as is known, strictly human qualities, the best evidence comes from studies of human subjects who have suffered injuries to these regions. One example is blindsight, in which people with lesions of their visual cortex are nonetheless able to respond to visual stimuli without being aware they have seen anything (Fox et al., 2020). Their behavioral responses are likely to be mediated through midbrain structures, as is the case with lower vertebrates, whereas their denial of sight suggests a predominantly cortical locus for visual awareness. Another example comes from lesions to the prefrontal cortex, which can rob individuals of the ability to generate long-term plans and express individual personalities (Miller et al., 2002). In this respect, it is noteworthy that the prefrontal cortex is so poorly developed in rodents that some believe it is absent; it is substantial in primates and largest in humans. The result that executive functions, which require entertaining multiple possibilities about the future and connecting them to a remembered past, are housed in a structure that is (nearly) primate-specific and largest in humans supports DeGrazia's view described above that autobiographical consciousness may be restricted to humans and perhaps their closest relatives.

A final question of great relevance to judging the potential of organoids for consciousness is the extent to which it depends on experience. The vertebrate central nervous system is initially assembled through a genetically determined plan, but this "rough draft" is then refined by experience as transduced into electrical neural activity (Sanes, 2021). Experience-dependent refinement occurs to some extent in all vertebrates, but appears to play a larger role in mammals than in other vertebrate classes, a larger role in primates than in other mammalian orders, and a larger role in the cortex than in subcortical structures. These relationships map well to what is known about the evolution and localization of consciousness. Thus, to the extent that higher levels of consciousness are housed in the human cortex, it is reasonable to imagine that they develop in an experience-dependent fashion. Moreover, to the extent that consciousness is defined in terms of subjective experience, it can occur only in the context of objective experience.

However, the capacity for consciousness is also a concern, as noted above, for pain, and here the need for experience is less clear. Complex neural circuitry can develop in the absence of external experience and even in the absence of electrical activity. In a classic experiment, a newt (axolotl) embryo was allowed to develop under conditions of paralysis and anesthesia, so that external stimulation and motor responses were eliminated. When the anesthetic was washed out, the tadpole swam away (Twitty, 1937). More recently, mice were studied in which synaptic transmission is prevented by mutation of key components of the neurotransmitter release apparatus. Again, the mice developed to term with brains relatively normal in structure, although they did not survive postnatally. In view of these results, it remains possible that the substrate for consciousness could form in the absence of experience even if experience were required for manifestation of consciousness.

It is generally agreed, however, that even the capacity for consciousness relies on complex patterns of circuitry that include multiple brain regions and connections between them. Given the current properties of organoids, the prospects for organoids achieving this level of complexity in the near future are remote. Likewise, transplants of human neural cells into nonhuman animals currently involve far too few cells to generate any capacity approaching consciousness. Chimeras, in contrast, raise distinct issues, which are considered in Chapter 3.

Emotion

Suffering can arise from sources other than physical pain—for example, sadness, fear, and anxiety. The neural bases of these emotions have been studied in at least three ways (Adolphs and Anderson, 2018; Anderson and Adolphs, 2014). First, a rich literature of human neuroimaging studies has pinpointed areas in the brain in which activity is correlated with negative emotions generally and with particular negative emotions specifically. These include such areas as prefrontal cortex, amygdala, and hypothalamus, together forming what is called the limbic system. Second, systems neuroscientists have used rodents, particularly genetically engineered mice, to trace neural circuits underlying such negative emotions as anxiety and fear. Third, an increasing number of studies have demonstrated responses in invertebrates (flies) that resemble, in several respects, states called aggression, fear, and anxiety in vertebrates.

Interpretation of work on emotions in rodents and especially invertebrates remains controversial because emotions are traditionally defined in terms of human behaviors accessible by introspection and self-report. Indeed, some experts argue against assuming that emotions of the sort recognized in humans are even present in other animals (LeDoux, 2012). Others, however, argue that "emotional behaviors are a class of behaviors that express internal emotion states. These emotion states exhibit certain general functional and adaptive properties that apply across all specific human emotions, such as fear or anger, as well as across phylogeny" (Anderson and Adolphs, 2014). Indeed, recent studies have even provided evidence that mice exhibit empathy: If one mouse is exposed to another mouse experiencing pain or fear, the observer will become more sensitive to painful or frightening stimuli (Klein and Gogolla, 2021). This transfer is related to a "theory of mind," once thought to be restricted to primates, in which an animal has some awareness of the experience of another animal. Based on this accumulation of evidence, it appears likely that rodents do have emotions. Therefore, assessment of emotional capacity in transplants or chimeras would have to be based not on acquisition of emotional responses, but rather on assessment of alterations in the emotional capability of the transplant or chimera compared with an unmanipulated host.

MEASURING CHARACTERISTICS OF HUMAN NEURAL ORGANOIDS, TRANSPLANTS, AND CHIMERAS

As research on human neural organoids, transplants, and chimeras proceeds, it will be increasingly important to devise methods for assessing their characteristics and capacities. These include consciousness, which, as discussed above, has resisted clear definition and is therefore difficult to assess. For other measures of complexity, however, some metrics exist.

Human Neural Organoids

At present, neural organoids lack complex and precise circuitry, are missing critical diversity among cell types, and do not include more than very limited representations of the multiple brain regions and long-range circuitry thought to underlie consciousness (Alves et al., 2019; Zirui et al., 2020). Thus, there is currently no objective basis for ascribing consciousness to organoids. Moreover, to the extent that consciousness requires experience and/or goal-directed behavior, it may be impossible for organoids to acquire consciousness in the foreseeable future. As organoid technology advances, however, assessment of their capacities may become more relevant, not only for purely scientific purposes but also to guide decisions about whether and under what circumstances they should or should not be used in research. The most reliable ways of assessing pain, consciousness, and related capacities are behavioral. It is possible that behavioral outputs could be inferred in cases in which human neural organoids are transplanted into the brains of host animals. For organoids maintained in culture, however, it is extremely unlikely that behavioral metrics will be feasible in the foreseeable future: Even when these organoids are connected to an output device, such as by innervating muscle cells, any outputs will be reflexive responses, which are inadequate for assessing consciousness or pain.

A feasible alternative will be to track how closely neural organoids and assembloids resemble actual brains. Anatomical, molecular, and physiological metrics can be assessed. Anatomical metrics include organoid size, number of cells, dendritic complexity of neurons, and synaptic connectivity. Immunohistochemical markers of specific cell classes or types can be applied to assess the degree to which neurons have differentiated (Albanese et al., 2020), the extent to which they are arranged into laminar or nuclear structures reminiscent of the brain, and the extent to which they display circuit motifs and activity dynamics characteristic of specific brain regions. Assessment can also include analyses of key glial types and properties, such as myelination, that are critical for normal neural function.

Molecular metrics, such as transcriptomic and epigenomic profiling using high-throughput single-cell or single-nucleus RNA-seq (scRNA-seq and snRNA-seq, respectively) (Quadrato et al., 2017), can be used to assess gene expression of many thousands of single cells per organoid. These methods are increasingly being applied to postmortem samples of developing and adult human brains, making it possible to compare gene expression patterns in organoids with those in vivo. From the comparison, one can assess the levels of differentiation and maturation of cells in the organoids, their diversification into distinct cell types, and the extent to which they resemble their in vivo counterparts. Proteomic and metabolomic measures can currently be made from whole organoids and are rapidly progressing to the single-cell level.

Physiological methods can be applied to assess patterns of neuronal activity and synaptic connectivity in neural organoids, comparing results with those obtained, for example, from human samples collected ex vivo. EEG (electroencephalogram) techniques have already been used in neural organoids (Trujillo et al., 2019). Physiological methods can be used to assess synaptic plasticity, which is thought to be the physical basis of learning and memory, and to determine whether synapses are regulated by such neuromodulatory substances as dopamine, norepinephrine, serotonin, and acetylcholine, which regulate plasticity and brain state. All of these methods are in common use and have already been applied to neural organoids to some extent, so technical challenges to their use are minimal.

At a higher level, the complexity of a neural system can be evaluated and even quantified by proposed physiological measures, such as the aforementioned PCI (Casali et al., 2013). This index is calculated from measurements of the complexity of an EEG response in both time and space following delivery of a pulse of transcranial magnetic stimulation to the brain. PCI levels have been shown to correlate with the level of consciousness in healthy humans (i.e., awake vs. sleep) and in patients who are anesthetized, minimally conscious, or comatose, indicating the PCI's potential utility in measuring consciousness. Thus far, the PCI has not been used across species to assess potentially informative differences, nor has it been applied to neural organoids. It has, however, been adapted for in vitro use to study connectivity and complexity in slices of mouse brain (D'Andola et al., 2018).

It should be noted, however, that these approaches cannot by themselves demonstrate the presence of consciousness. It is more useful to think of these characteristics as being necessary but not sufficient for consciousness. As the cell types, circuits, signaling mechanisms, and regional specializations of neural organoids become increasingly brain-like, concerns about conscious states will need to be reconsidered.

Human Neural Cell Transplants and Chimeras

Most of the tests described above for neural organoids can also be applied to transplants and chimeras. A critical difference, however, is that behavioral tests can be used to determine whether any capacities of animals with human neural cell transplants or chimeric animals differ from those of their unmanipulated counterparts. Cognitive capabilities can be measured with assays for learning and memory that are well established in animal models (such as those used by Han and colleagues [2013]). A promising recent advance is the introduction of methods for capturing and quantifying behavior at high spatial and temporal resolution (Mathis and Mathis, 2020; Mathis et al., 2018; Oikarinen et al., 2019; Wiltschko et al., 2020). These new methods can identify discrete, elementary behavioral motifs that are stitched together in different ways to generate more sophisticated, goal-directed behaviors. They come closer than traditional methods to harmonizing the scales of behavioral and physiological measures, and therefore improve the ability to assess possible consequences of augmenting nonhuman brains with human neurons.

Researchers have also developed behavioral metrics for other types of awareness or emotional capabilities that range from whether nonhuman animals feel pain (e.g., learned avoidance of painful stimuli) to tests of self-awareness (e.g., a mirror test to determine whether an animal recognizes itself in a mirror [Anderson and Gallup, 2015]; see Figure 2-5), metacognition (Smith, 2010), and capacity for empathy (de Waal and Preston, 2017; Klein and Gogolla, 2021). However, many of these assays can be difficult to design and interpret because nonhuman animals may not express these traits in a way that is obvious to humans (de Waal, 2019). In view of the difficulty of measuring consciousness directly, Pennartz and colleagues (2019) have proposed an alternative approach, based on assessment of multiple qualities they call "indicators" of consciousness, none individually decisive but highly suggestive in the aggregate (see, e.g., Edelman et al., 2005; Seth et al., 2005). They include goal-directed behavior, the presence of circuits that mediate multimodal integration, episodic memory, susceptibility to illusions, and specific visuospatial behaviors. Going forward, it will be essential to reach agreement on an operational definition of consciousness and on acceptable methods for assessing its presence. However difficult to attain, this community consensus will provide a basis for oversight as transplant and chimera research progresses.

3

Ethical Concerns

Research involving human neural organoids, transplants, and chimeras has an ultimate goal of preventing and treating the great suffering caused by serious neurological and psychiatric conditions for which no effective treatment is available. Current models for such diseases, which are essential for discovering mechanisms and testing therapeutic interventions, have significant limitations. As explained in Chapter 2, human neural organoids, transplants, and chimeras provide new models for such conditions and may lead to new knowledge about brain development and function, the discovery of disease mechanisms, new therapeutic targets, and better screening of potential new treatments.

As the power of these research models advances, however, so, too, do the ethical concerns they raise. Some of these concerns, such as ensuring the welfare of research animals and obtaining appropriate consent for the use of human tissues, also apply to many other areas of research, but may require special consideration for research with human neural organoids, cell transplants, and chimeras. Other concerns are more specific to these research models. One such concern is the possibility of altering the capacities or consciousness of a research animal in ways that may blur the lines between human beings and nonhuman animals. This concern becomes particularly acute when nonhuman primates are used as animal hosts.

Chapter 2 presents the science behind these models and describes the challenges of measuring and monitoring such characteristics and capacities in human neural organoids, transplants, and chimeras. These capacities are rudimentary at present, but because the field is developing quickly, it is important to consider both current ethical concerns and those that might be raised by enhanced capacities in the future. The current chapter first looks at ethical issues common to human neural organoids, transplants, and chimeras, and then at issues specific to human neural transplants and chimeras or to neural organoids. Chapter 4 considers oversight and regulatory mechanisms that may address some of these concerns.

ISSUES COMMON TO ALL THREE MODELS

Ethical issues common to human neural organoids, transplants, and chimeras include (1) the ethical value of relieving human suffering and disease, (2) concerns about encroachment on divine roles, and (3) ethical issues related to human donors of biological materials.

Ethical Value of Relieving Human Suffering and Disease

A main justification for carrying out research, both basic and translational, with human neural organoids, transplants, and chimeras is that it will help in the discovery of new ways to understand and treat neurological and psychiatric disorders, which, as discussed previously, cause immense suffering and for which treatments are ineffective or lacking.

Given the complexity of the human brain and the particularly human nature of many key symptoms of these disorders, especially psychiatric disorders, animal and cell culture models of the types currently used to investigate diseases of other organs and tissues are valuable but inadequate. For example, mouse models of age-related neurodegenerative diseases fail to capture key features because the diseases typically strike humans in their 60s and 70s, whereas mice live for only 2 or 3 years. Likewise, behavioral disorders such as autism, depression, and schizophrenia involve alterations in emotional and cognitive capacities that may not exist in mice and may involve brain areas, such as prefrontal cortex, that are rudimentary in mice (Feng et al., 2020).

For many people, there are strong moral reasons to pursue this research to relieve human suffering and treat human diseases. The rationale is rooted in the widely shared values of preventing harm to human beings, advancing their well-being, and acting with compassion toward people in need (Parker, 2020). Acquisition of knowledge is also often seen as an ethical good. These benefits are not absolute, however, and must be weighed against other ethical values discussed next.

Concerns about Encroachment on Divine Roles

Some commentators invoke the phrase "playing God" to indicate opposition to biotechnology, such as research with human neural organoids, transplants, and chimeras, with the implication that human activities should not infringe on the role of a deity as the creator of life. Many others, however, believe that this injunction does not preclude the treatment of serious human diseases (Hauerwas, 1986). One scholar believes that it is more typical of Christians to believe that they are called to intentionally "play God in the correct way" or "play God as God plays God" by, for example, healing the sick (Verhey, 1995). Similarly, many Jewish and Christian thinkers view human intervention in nature as completing God's unfinished creation (Cole-Turner, 1993; Loike and Tendler, 2008).[1] They argue that since human beings were created by God with reason and intellect, God allows, encourages, and enjoins human beings to use their capacities to improve the earth, heal human disease, and relieve human suffering. Creation in this view is a continuous process, with humans being cocreators of the universe with God (Cole-Turner, 1993).

Some believe that nonhuman animals as well as humans were created by a deity and have their own purpose and nature—their own telos—that should be respected (Comosy and Kopp, 2014). This view is not, however, incompatible with the idea that human beings can be justified in utilizing other species. Speakers and writers representing several faith traditions and secular beliefs generally agree that humans are permitted to use nonhuman animals for the benefit of humanity, including in work, for food, and in well-justified research projects (Comosy and Kopp, 2014; Loike and Tendler, 2008; Tlili, 2018). However, they also agree that humans should be stewards of nonhuman animals and should not cause them to suffer needlessly or treat them cruelly. The committee notes, however, that beliefs and interpretations vary both within and among faith traditions, and people will differ in what aspects of human neural organoid, transplant, and chimera research, if any, cross an unacceptable line between the roles of a deity and humans.

Ethical Issues Related to Human Donors of Biological Materials

For research described in this report, the starting points are most often stem cells that can be treated to differentiate into neural precursors and then into neurons or glia. In some cases these are embryonic stem cells (ESCs) derived from early embryos, but increasingly they are somatic cells that can be reprogrammed to generate induced pluripotent stem cells (iPSCs). iPSCs are usually derived from skin biopsies as shown in Figure 2-3, but can also be generated from other tissues, blood, or even the few cells present in urine. Some research uses neural tissue that is resected during surgery or obtained postmortem, tissues that would otherwise be discarded.

There is broad agreement on the need to respect humans who provide biological materials used to generate human neural organoids, transplants, or chimeras. An ethical concern might arise when cells used to generate these models are derived from people who did not know that such research was being carried out, did not give permission for use of their tissues for this purpose, or would not have consented had they known. Respect for persons who provide tissues for such research plays out differently for new collection of biospecimens and for use of existing biospecimens.

---

[1] John Loike, Columbia University, presentation to committee, October 29, 2020, virtual meeting.

Collection of New Biospecimens for Research

As described in Chapter 4, federal regulations for the protection of human research subjects mandate informed consent before researchers can collect fresh biological materials for research, whether by collecting tissue left over from surgery and biopsies, or by extracting tissue specifically for research. The ethical rationale is the need to respect donors as persons and to protect their liberty interests in being free of unwanted excision of tissue. (As noted earlier, this report uses the term "donor" rather than the longer and more cumbersome phrase "persons from whom biospecimens used in research are obtained, although they may not have made a conscious decision to do so.")

For consent to be informed, the donor needs to be told about the research studies to be carried out and the risks entailed in obtaining the specimens. If human neural organoid, transplant, or chimera research is contemplated when new biospecimens are obtained, the donor should be so informed. However, because future research uses of biospecimens cannot always be envisioned in advance, consent forms for biopsies or surgical procedures commonly include a sentence granting broad permission to conduct unspecified research on materials that are not needed for clinical care. Some consent forms separate consent for surgery from consent for future research on the removed tissue to make clear that patients may have the clinical procedure without agreeing to research on their excised tissue. Later in this chapter is a discussion of debates over whether such broad consent should or should not be viewed as sufficient when cells are used to generate human neural organoids or chimeras.

Use of Existing Biospecimens for Research

Persons who provided existing biospecimens need to be respected when those specimens are used in research. Their privacy and autonomy are protected by removing specified identifiers from the biomaterials, prohibiting attempts to reidentify them, and not carrying out research that is contrary to the conditions of the original consent.

Research may be carried out without consent in several circumstances. With existing specimens, the overt identifiers can be removed so that the identities of the donors can no longer be readily ascertained. Consistent with common usage, this report refers to such biospecimens as "deidentified." As discussed in Chapter 4, under current federal regulations, such deidentified existing materials can be used in research without obtaining additional consent because the persons who provided the biological materials are no longer human subjects; therefore, Part A of the Federal Policy for the Protection of Human Subjects (generally called the Common Rule and described in Chapter 4) does not apply to them. The underlying ethical rationale for this regulatory provision is that using a leftover biospecimen for research provides a social good compared with discarding the specimen, and the risks to the donor are minimal because the specimen has already been removed from the donor's body, and confidentiality will be protected. An additional rationale is that people should not retain control over biological materials that are already outside their body and that they have given away voluntarily or abandoned (Charo, 2006).

A common example is the use of leftover tubes of blood for research after clinical tests ordered by the treating physician have been completed, and explicit identifying information has been removed from the biospecimen. Generally, there is no written informed consent for "routine" clinical blood tests, and even oral consent is often perfunctory; consent is implied when the patient presents to the clinical laboratory for the test and makes no objection to the phlebotomy. However, ethical views and institutional and public policies can change. In 2007, for example, Vanderbilt Medical Center started a deidentified repository of genomic sequencing data extracted from leftover clinical specimens matched with electronic health records. Biospecimens and records were placed into the repository unless patients chose to opt out. The medical center offered the option to opt out even though it was not required to do so, because the creators of that resource believed it was important to allow some choice. In 2015, the medical center's policy changed to an opt-in policy. It began to require signed affirmative consent from the patient to participate in genomic studies using biomaterials and clinical data from which identifiers had been removed, consistent with a new National Institutes of Health (NIH) policy (Vanderbilt University Medical Center, 2015). An ongoing challenge for biorepositories is that the increasing availability of genomic, transcriptomic, and other information about individuals is making true deidentification more difficult; this issue is discussed in Chapter 4.

There may be a disparity in some situations between what is legally permitted by the Common Rule and what is considered ethically acceptable. For example, "pinprick" blood samples (blood spots) are routinely obtained from newborns in the United States to screen for congenital diseases. These archived materials have been a valuable resource for public health research for many years. After the samples and accompanying data have been processed so that the identities of the babies can no longer be readily ascertained, secondary research is permitted without consent in all but a few states. In response to parental concerns, however, Texas now offers parents an opportunity to opt out of such research, and Michigan now requires affirmative consent.

Another example of requiring specific consent for a particular type of research with materials originally collected for clinical care is the NIH requirements for funding human embryonic stem cell (hESC) research (NIH, 2016). For research using hESC lines derived after 2009, consent forms to donate the embryos must explicitly state that the embryos would be used to derive hESCs for research and describe what would happen to the embryos in that derivation; a broad consent to donate embryos "for research" would not suffice.

For deidentified biological materials already collected and available in tissue banks, specific informed consent for use of cells to generate human neural organoids, transplants, or chimeras typically has not been obtained; rather, consent has been obtained for broad use in research, or the identities of the donors of the biospecimens could no longer be readily ascertained. Under federal regulations, such biospecimens can be used to generate iPSCs without further consent, and the iPSCs can then be used to generate human neural organoids, transplants, or chimeras. Of note, the derivation and use of iPSCs render moot the objections that some people have to the derivation of hESCs, which requires destruction of early embryos.

Whatever the current requirements for informed consent, it is likely that some donors of biological materials may not want those materials to be used for such projects and would object to such use if they knew about it (Grady et al., 2015; Streiffer, 2008). Prospectively, it would be feasible to obtain specific informed consent for the collection of fresh tissue for production of iPSCs from which human neural organoids, transplants, and chimeras can be generated. However, logistical problems could arise in managing tissues and databases of thousands and even millions of samples, each with its own list of permissible experiments. Alternatively, tissue banks could institute review and governance procedures for determining whether future research projects fall outside the scope of the initial consent for research and whether the project might conflict with the values of the donors (Grady et al., 2015).

For existing biospecimens, requiring specific consent for such research might be considered ethically problematic for several reasons. First, some question whether donors of biological materials have an ethical right to control materials they have already given away voluntarily or abandoned (Charo, 2006; Rao, 2016). Second, in some cases, there are strong scientific reasons to use biological materials already collected even if the donors did not provide specific informed consent for human neural organoid, transplant, or chimera research. Some cell lines have been well characterized using many methods over a long period; redoing this foundational research with newly collected tissues would require considerable time and funding. For very rare diseases, moreover, it may not be feasible to identify and recruit new donors. Trying to recontact the original donors to obtain specific informed consent is sometimes impossible, could impede important research, and might not be welcomed by some donors. Policy in this area is actively debated in an effort to strike the right balance between anticipating and respecting donor preferences in sensitive areas and developing new therapeutics for serious diseases in a timely manner.

Consent in Groups That Have Suffered Health Disparities and Discrimination

Use of human cells to generate human neural organoids, transplants, and chimeras could elicit mistrust in such groups as African Americans that suffer health disparities, unequal treatment, and discrimination (IOM, 2003). Public awareness of past research abuses, such as in the Henrietta Lacks case, could fuel this concern (see, e.g., Skloot, 2010). In that case, cancerous tissue was removed during clinical care of Henrietta Lacks, a Black woman, and given to researchers to create cell lines without telling the patient or family that this was being done. When the surgery was carried out in 1951, there were no federal regulations for human subjects research. The HeLa cell line derived from the tissue has been widely shared among researchers and "played an extraordinary role in scientific research," enabling many important medical advances and generating substantial profits for some who used it (see Jones et al., 1971; Wolinetz and Collins, 2020). In 1971, Lacks' name was published in a medical article on the eponymous HeLa cell line. In 2013, researchers published her complete genomic sequence online, which violated investigator responsibility for release of genomic sequences and for stewardship of sensitive data (Greely and Cho, 2013). In response to concerns about this case, NIH and the Lacks family held discussions and agreed that family members would serve on a data access committee for future use of her cells, and that all publications using this cell line would acknowledge her and her family.

Empirical studies provide evidence that the Henrietta Lacks case is salient today for persons from minority backgrounds. In a 2019 study, focus groups were convened with persons from five ethnic and racial groups regarding the collection of biospecimens and electronic health record data for research (Lee et al., 2019). The article reporting the study findings was titled "I don't want to be Henrietta Lacks." The researchers found that "many participants across our five racial and ethnic groups cited the case of Henrietta Lacks as a cautionary tale when discussing potential risks associated with biospecimens." Respondents associated a range of concerns with the case in response to open-ended questions, including loss of control of the self, unfair profits to companies from samples of unsuspecting patients, and limited ability to conceive of potential future research.

Strengthening informed consent could be a component of an approach designed to build trust and increase participation of minority communities currently underrepresented in research. On the 100th birthday of Henrietta Lacks, leaders at NIH (Wolinetz and Collins, 2020) and the editors of *Nature* (Nature Editorials, 2020) called for a revision of ethical and regulatory standards for research with human biospecimens to require consent for use in research. "A genuine culture of respect for research participants demands that they be asked to agree to use of their biospecimens, regardless of identifiability" (Wolinetz and Collins, 2020).

Indigenous peoples might object to biological materials collected for one purpose being used in deidentified form in other research that they would not have consented to had they known about it. For example, the Havasupai tribe objected when materials collected under a consent for research on diabetes, which is highly prevalent in the tribe, were later used for projects on the genetic basis of schizophrenia and inbreeding because such research could stigmatize the tribe or violate cultural values (Garrison, 2013). To settle a lawsuit, Arizona State University, whose researchers conducted the disputed studies, apologized; returned the remaining samples to the tribe; made a monetary payment; and agreed to work with the tribe on health, education, and economic development (Mello and Wolf, 2010).

These concerns among ethnic and racial groups regarding the use of biological materials for certain types of research without consent have not specifically addressed research with human neural organoids, transplants, or chimeras. Nonetheless, they resemble concerns that may arise in such research. It will therefore be important to engage these communities in discussions about such research to identify and address particular sensitivities.

Other strategies can also help overcome mistrust and increase minority participation in research. The federally funded All of Us project, which studies relationships among genetics, lifestyle, environment, and health outcomes, is making a determined effort to increase inclusion and minority enrollment (Mapes et al., 2020). The Jackson Heart Study, a community-based cohort study evaluating the etiology of cardiovascular, renal, and respiratory diseases among African Americans, has successfully recruited participants and followed them for 20 years. The research included genomic sequencing of participants, a type of research in which African Americans had historically participated at very low rates (Popejoy and Fullerton, 2016). This study has a strong commitment to community education and outreach to promote healthy lifestyles and reduce cardiovascular risk, research training programs for college and graduate students, and high school science and math enrichment programs to prepare and encourage underrepresented minority students to pursue biomedical careers. This sustained community engagement has enabled an important long-term study in a group whose medical care has suffered from a relative paucity of research on diseases that disproportionately afflict them.

ISSUES SPECIFIC TO HUMAN NEURAL ORGANOIDS, TRANSPLANTS, AND CHIMERAS

Ethical issues raised specifically by human neural organoids, transplants, and chimeras include (1) concerns related to distinctions between humans and other animals, (2) concerns about animal welfare and rights, (3) concerns about consciousness and enhanced capacities, and (4) concerns related to the use of nonhuman primates.

Concerns Related to Distinctions between Humans and Other Animals

Several concerns specific to neural transplants and chimeras revolve around a distinction between humans and other animals that is widely held across cultures (De Cruz and De Smedt, 2016). This distinction may be based on interpretations of religious texts and teachings: for instance, that humans were created by God as different from other animals, or were created in God's image and thus have a higher status than other animals (Loike and Tendler, 2008). In a secular context, this distinction arises from the common-sense notion that "nature" made humans different from other animals. Summarizing these views, Robert and Baylis (2003) suggest that there are moral if not biological boundaries between species that are common in public opinion, whether or not they correspond to biological distinctions (see also Baylis and Robert, 2007). From a perspective that need not involve religious views, some ethicists believe that each nonhuman animal species has a distinctive nature or kind that should be respected by humans and allowed to flourish in accordance with its own telos or end.

Every culture has foundational cultural distinctions, which people within that culture believe to a greater or lesser extent. Blurring these distinctions results in fascination and repugnance; many cultures have a fascination with mythical chimeras that violate the human/animal distinction. By eroding a foundational cultural distinction between humans and other animals, human neural cell transplants and chimeras might create "moral confusion," which is, for some people, accompanied by a sense of repugnance (Robert and Baylis, 2003). For instance, some might feel revulsion at the possibility of a human brain being trapped inside an animal's body. Beyond the intrinsic reasons to avoid mixing humans and animals, people who write about "moral confusion" are typically concerned that such confusion would lead some people to think of humans differently and treat them worse—more like nonhuman animals are treated. Others might be concerned about enhancing the capacities of animals to turn them into a "service" species that could be exploited by human beings. In contrast, still others hope that breaking down the human/animal distinction would lead to treating nonhuman animals better (Greely, 2020).

Immediate Negative Reactions to Perceived Violations of Distinctions between Humans and Nonhuman Animals

Kass (1997) forcefully argued for the moral value of feelings of repugnance toward situations that violate the distinction between human beings and nonhuman animals and threaten human dignity:

> Revulsion is not an argument; and some of yesterday's repugnances are today calmly accepted though, one must add, not always for the better. In crucial cases, however, repugnance is the emotional expression of deep wisdom, beyond reason's power fully to articulate it. Can anyone really give an argument fully adequate to the horror which is father-daughter incest (even with consent), or having sex with animals, or mutilating a corpse, or eating human flesh...? Would anybody's failure to give full rational justification for his or her revulsion at these practices make that revulsion ethically suspect? Not at all.

Such immediate reactions of repugnance and disgust are commonly if inelegantly called a "yuck" response. These reactions should not be dismissed: They represent views that are plausible, deeply felt, and consistent with core values. Moreover, they have had important policy impact on many topics, including genetically engineered food (Scott et al., 2018), wastewater recycling (Miller, 2012), control of infectious diseases (Curtis, 2011), and human reproductive cloning (Kass, 1997). On the other hand, disgust may also lead to shunning, stigmatization, and prejudice (Curtis, 2011). With regard to the topics of this report, human neural organoids, transplants, and chimeras may elicit "yuck" responses (Devolder et al., 2020; Smith, 2020).

Culturally approved repugnance may shift dramatically over time, examples being the overturning of legal support for school segregation and bans on racial intermarriage in the mid-20th century. Thus, a consensus view is that repugnance should invite inquiry, reflection, and respectful dialogue, but not unquestioning acceptance (Schmidt, 2008; Smits, 2006). Most people readily accept the idea of using nonhuman animal tissues, such as heart valves or cartilage, for transplantation, but clearly there is some degree of admixture that will violate people's intuitive moral sense, and neural tissue may well be problematic for many. Further inquiry and discussion can illuminate the point at which the technologies discussed in this report violate common feelings of repugnance or foundational distinctions. In terms of developing science policy and public policy regarding human neural organoids, transplants, and chimeras, there may be lessons to be learned from experiences cited above, such as those involving genetically engineered food or reproductive cloning (Miller, 2012; Scott et al., 2018).

Other writers have attempted to analyze the origins of these reactions. Rozin traces the biological and cultural evolution of disgust, whose triggers vary through history and across cultures (Rozin and Haidt, 2013; Rozin, 2015). Curtis (2011) shows how disgust evolved to motivate avoidance of infectious diseases. Niemela (2011) argues that "people have certain automatic and quick cognitive tendencies routinely used for categorizing and reasoning about living nature." (p. 272). He continues, "As the cognitive tendencies routinely applied to the explanation of biological world are violated, an emotional response of fear, disgust and of something unnatural being underway is easily provoked." (p. 267).

Importantly, faith traditions vary in the implications they draw for animal welfare and status from the distinction—whether clear or blurred—between humans and other species. For some, the distinction leads to a strong elevation in the worth of humans over nonhuman animals, with a consequent decreased regard for animal welfare. In other faith traditions, by contrast, nonhuman animals were created by God on the same day as human beings and participate in the afterlife (Tlili, 2018). Such views would require that human beings act as stewards of other animals and give greater consideration to their interests and welfare.

Concerns Related to Attributes of Chimeric Animals

Another concern is that a nonhuman animal that received a human neural cell transplant or a chimera could become human if it obtained enough "human-like" capacities. There is no single definition of what it means to be human, but rather several conceptions that are not mutually exclusive (Evans, 2016). One traditional

Jewish and Christian definition is that humans are made in the image of God and have a soul and free will (Loike and Tendler, 2008; Niederauer, 2010).[2] The importance of free will and other capacities can also be framed in secular terms. A second view is that human beings are conceived through the fertilization of human gametes, gestated in a woman's womb, and born of a human mother. A third, biological view is that genes determine which entities are human. A fourth conception is based on capabilities that are believed to confer moral status, such as self-awareness (Evans, 2016) or high-level consciousness.

Yet another common definition of a human depends on appearance and behavior (Greely, 2020). By this criterion, neural transplants or chimeras that appear human, have a visible human feature, or act like a human would be particularly unsettling (Katsyri et al., 2015). Several years ago, a furor developed when tissue was attached to a rodent in a way that allowed it to differentiate into a structure vaguely resembling a human pinna (outer ear) (Cao et al., 1997; Hugo, 2017). A public consultation in the UK found that people were particularly concerned with "cellular or genetic modifications which could result in nonhuman animals with aspects of human-like appearance (skin type, limb or facial structure) or characteristics, such as speech" (Academy of Medical Sciences, 2011). In short, given this multiplicity of conceptions, it is helpful in discussions of ethical issues to specify which are or are not being referenced.

In some of these conceptions, human-nonhuman animal neural transplants and chimeras involving the brain arouse stronger concerns relative to those involving other organs because many of the capacities associated with higher moral status, such as consciousness, complex problem solving, self-awareness, and emotions, are "located" in the brain. From a more introspective view, the brain more than any other organ is believed to define who a person is. As the physical instantiation of characteristics that many people commonly associate with their humanness and individuality, the brain evokes greater concern relative to other organs.

Importantly, although these different definitions of "human" arise from different ethical perspectives, it is possible for people to reach agreement on specific issues and problems, even though they do not agree on the reasons for their common conclusions (Jonsen and Toulmin, 1988). This report aims to reflect how adherents of different positions would present their arguments. The committee was not asked to make recommendations on which views are most convincing; indeed, trying to do so would be fraught because positions often build from deeply held individual beliefs.

Concerns Related to Potential Capacities of Chimeric Animals

People concerned about nonhuman animals developing human-like attributes from any of a variety of ethical perspectives might believe that even the *possibil-*

---

[2] Charles Camosy, Fordham University, presentation to committee, October 30, 2020, virtual meeting.

ity that such animals would develop is to be avoided and oppose research that could lead this possibility to become reality. From a precautionary perspective, they would argue that in cases of uncertainty, it is advisable to close off areas of research that could lead to such troubling outcomes. There are many versions of this so-called "slippery-slope" argument. "The common feature of the different forms is the contention that once the first step is taken on a slippery slope the subsequent steps follow inexorably, whether for logical reasons, psychological reasons, or to avoid arbitrariness in 'drawing a line' between a person's actions" (Young, 2020). In the specific case of neural transplantation and chimera research, the slippery slope concern is that if small increments in mental capacities develop in transplants or chimeras, there will be no logical point at which the research should be stopped, or it may not be possible later to institute policies to block research that could result in nonhuman animals with unacceptable human capabilities.

If barriers cannot be set far down the slope to protect against the ethically objectionable bottom, some would say that researchers should not step onto the slope at all. The difficulty with this view is that a strict application of precautionary principles would close off entirely the possibility of gaining new knowledge that could result in treatments to relieve suffering in patients with serious neurological and psychiatric diseases. To gain the benefits of such research, it is necessary to balance its prospective benefits with its risks. Such a balance could take the form of a tiered approach to oversight, with the final tier—research that should not proceed at this time—acting as a barrier on the slope. When the science began to approach that limit, a greater understanding of the science and the associated ethics could allow a more strongly justified limit to be set. Chapter 4 describes current guidelines for neural cell transplant and chimera research that represent an attempt to instantiate this approach.

Concerns Related to Human Gametes in Chimeric Animals

It is possible that in the course of generating human neural chimeras, some human cells could populate the germline—that is, become gametes. In this case, objections to chimerism would likely be far greater than if the human cells contributed only to somatic tissues. For those who see humans and nonhuman animals as created distinctly by God, the idea of creating nonhuman animals that could pass a human genome to future generations is more disturbing than that of creating animals that could not do so. Reproduction also has particular significance because it usually begins with an intimate and private encounter and results in the transmission of familial lineage. The idea of nonhuman animals with human gametes might lead people to fear that such an animal could give birth to a monster or that these important personal and social aspects of reproduction would be undermined. While such a phenomenon would not logically blur the human/nonhuman distinction itself, it would blur notions of the role of human female gestation.

In practice, it is unlikely that cells of human origin could become competent gametes in a nonhuman animal because of the multiple stringent biological restrictions used by each species to protect its germline. Moreover, current NIH guidelines prohibit the mating of any nonhuman animals in which human gametes could be formed (NIH, 2009), but this prohibition might provide scant comfort to some concerned people. Perhaps most useful would be to engineer human cells to prevent them absolutely from developing into gametes when used in chimeric animals, an option made feasible by available knowledge of genes required for gametogenesis. These engineered stem cells could be used—indeed, their use could be mandated—for the generation of chimeras.

Concerns about Animal Welfare and Rights

Some perspectives on animal ethics hold that nonhuman animals have their own inherent value quite apart from the benefits humans can derive from them. In this view, animals ought to be treated as the kinds of creatures they are—their intrinsic nature or telos should be respected—and they should not be treated as mere tools or things to be used for the benefit of humans (Carbone, 2019). Some animal rights advocates argue for banning all animal research, as well as killing of animals, whether it be for food or in research (Gruen, 2017).

In contrast, many people who believe that nonhuman animals have interests and deserve respect nonetheless accept their use for research directed toward the ultimate goal of relieving human suffering, as long as the research is well justified; harm to animals is minimized; and the physical, social, and psychological needs of the animals are met. Indeed, at least one prominent proponent of animal rights and vegetarianism endorses animal research under some circumstances, such as to relieve severe human suffering when there is a lack of alternative approaches (Crawley, 2006). This balancing of countervailing ethical values is the basis of current oversight of research involving animals in the United States.

In the United States, a major ethical framework to guide oversight of research with animals is known as the Three R's. The Three R's call on researchers to: *r*educe the number of animals, *r*eplace animals with other experimental models, and *r*efine methods for alleviating or minimizing pain and distress consistent with the scientific aims of the research (see Table 3-1). In addition, the U.S. government requires compliance with the Guide for the Care and Use of Laboratory Animals, which states that those overseeing animal research are "obliged to weigh the objectives of the study against potential animal welfare concerns" (NRC, 2011).

The definitions of the Three R's are evolving, with an increased focus on improving understanding of the impact of animal welfare on scientific outcomes. Moreover, there have been recent proposals to expand the Three R's to provide a more comprehensive ethical framework (Beauchamp and DeGrazia, 2020). These proposals include placing additional emphasis on animal welfare, including the

TABLE 3-1 The Three R's

	Standard	Contemporary
Replacement	Methods which avoid or replace the use of animals	Accelerating the development and use of models and tools, based on the latest science and technologies, to address important scientific questions without the use of animals
Reduction	Methods which minimize the number of animals used per experiment	Appropriately designed and analyzed animal experiments that are robust and reproducible, and truly add to the knowledge base
Refinement	Methods which minimize animal suffering and improve welfare	Advancing animal welfare by exploiting the latest *in vivo* technologies and by improving understanding of the impact of welfare on scientific outcomes

SOURCE: Margaret Landi, GlaxoSmithKline, presentation to committee, October 30, 2020, virtual meeting.

obligation to meet animals' basic needs, such as nutritious food, safe shelter, species-appropriate housing, companionship, and opportunities for stimulation and exercise. Other proposed additions focus on limiting harm to animal subjects and limiting potential suffering to that justified by the prospect of benefit to humans and required to address the research question. The expanded framework is still developing and more explicit discussion and analysis of how to balance the benefits of research to humans with the harms to research animals will be important to its further development.

Although the Three R's formulation provides only a conceptual outline rather than practical guidance, a rich reservoir of expertise—including veterinarians, animal caretakers in research facilities, and animal ethologists and experts in animal behavior—can be called on to address more practical concerns (ASP, 2020; IPS, 2007; Weatherall, 2006). Research veterinarians in particular have expertise and experience in identifying whether an animal is suffering distress and if so, how to provide relief in the context of the research. Importantly, they generally report to the institution rather than the researchers, so they can provide a view that is less likely to be unduly influenced by a commitment to specific research objectives.

Animal rights advocates believe if research with nonhuman animals is permitted, the animals have a right to what is necessary for them to flourish as the kind of beings they are. According to this perspective, the researcher's obligation to provide appropriate living conditions is similar to the requirements of the animal welfare perspective described earlier in this section. In some cases, however, animal rights advocates might object to some research that would be permitted by a balancing of countervailing values described earlier—for example, objecting to the creation of chimeric animals as violating their telos or nature.

Some countries have adopted principles for the treatment of animals broader than those that underlie U.S. regulations, incorporating animal rights perspectives that go well beyond the Three R's. Directive 2010/63/EU in the European

Union states that animals have an intrinsic value that must be respected and that animals should always be treated as sentient creatures.[3] The Swiss constitution and Animal Welfare Law includes the concept of "animal dignity," which grants animals a moral value irrespective of their sentience, and recognizes the need to protect an animal's inherent worth beyond avoidance of physical pain, injury, and anxiety (Bollinger, 2016).[4] Some animal rights advocates object to research conducted even under such an "expanded Three R's" framework. Many of the most restrictive policies for great apes were influenced by the Great Ape Project, which calls for chimpanzees, gorillas, bonobos, and orangutans to be accorded the same basic rights as human beings, including the rights to life, freedom, and not being tortured (GAP, n.d.). Additionally, animal rights advocates commonly have more concerns about the research use of higher nonhuman primates in research than about the use of other animals, such as mice. Issues specific to nonhuman primates are discussed below.

Finally, as human neural chimeras are developed to better recapitulate human disease, research animals may show altered capacities or behaviors similar to human symptoms of the disease, which may heighten concerns about animal welfare. Depending on the model, these behaviors could include changes in socializing, exploratory behavior, or eating patterns; increased anxiety; or other signs of distress. As noted above, veterinarians, animal caregivers, behavioral biologists, and ethologists can play a crucial role in identifying for institutional animal use and care committees (IACUCs) and researchers those behaviors in research animals that differ from the typical behavior of the individual animal or the species and how their care can be modified to take into account their changed needs and capacities (IACUCs are discussed in Chapter 4).[5] Animals in these studies may need to be treated differently from other research animals of their species that have not undergone such interventions. Overall, ensuring animal welfare requires mitigating any distress, which may include making appropriate changes to the care of animals (for example, changes in caging, environment, feeding, or enrichment) or to the research protocol, provided this can be done without undermining the justified aims of the research or the validity of the research data (Carbone, 2019).

Concerns about Consciousness and Enhanced Capacities

As noted earlier, the possibility of generating consciousness, suffering, or markedly enhanced cognitive capacities in human neural organoids, transplants, or chimeras has generated ethical concerns. The presence of or potential for con-

---

[3] EU Directive 2010/63/EU, Recital 12.
[4] Animal Welfare Act 7 U.S.C. § 2131–2159, A.S. 2965 (2008) § 3a.
[5] Megan Albertelli, Stanford University, presentation to the committee, August 11, 2020, virtual meeting. Margaret Landi, GlaxoSmithKline, presentation to the committee, October 30, 2020, virtual meeting.

sciousness is, for many, an important determination of the moral status that should be accorded to living entities (Van Gulick, 2018). The concept of consciousness is reviewed in Chapter 2. That discussion suggests that the development of consciousness would be extremely unlikely and perhaps impossible in the neural organoids currently being developed for research, but also notes the difficulty of defining consciousness and the practical impediments to assessing the possibility of enhanced consciousness in animals. The current failure to generate viable human-nonhuman chimeras renders consideration of their consciousness moot. However, if such chimeras are generated in the future, heightened consciousness or capabilities cannot be ruled out. If detected in a chimeric animal, they would surely change how human beings regard the animal and increase the obligations owed to the animal. Likewise, it will be imperative to assess the capacity of such chimeras to experience pain, and to ask whether that capacity differs from that of the unmanipulated host species. Finally, the experiences of consciousness and pain are not the only causes for concern. For many other thinkers, the mere capacity to suffer or acquire consciousness is all that is needed to impose an obligation to refrain from experimentation.

It will be important to clarify which specific enhancements to consciousness or capacities might increase the obligations of humans toward chimeric animals. People have several distinct concerns. First, consciousness may be thought to raise the moral status of the research animal or organoid and justify more research safeguards, oversight, and restrictions. Second, for some people, the possibility that the entity might have or develop enhanced consciousness is itself an ethical concern based on considerations detailed above, such as altering the nature of the animal, blurring natural distinctions between species, undermining human dignity, or eliciting repugnance. Third, research that causes an animal to experience pain, particularly pain beyond what it would usually experience, could be regarded as failing to respect the animal and its nature. For some, the capacity of animals to suffer generates obligations for humans to refrain from harming them. The committee notes that there is a range of views on such issues and on how to balance obligations toward animals with other ethical obligations, such as relieving severe suffering in human beings.

Additional ethical concerns about heightened consciousness or capabilities in a chimeric animal arise in people who hold that human beings have a special moral status. For some, these concerns are based on Jewish or Christian religious beliefs that human beings were created in the image of God and should act as stewards for creation. Others have nonreligious reasons for such concerns, which may be based on a concept of human dignity or of natural boundaries between species. Several basic capacities in addition to consciousness have been claimed to be uniquely human, including empathy, altruism, imitative learning (replicating a model's behavior rather than seeking alternative methods to achieve a goal), joint attention (a creature and social partner simultaneously attend to a stimulus and are aware of the shared attention), having a theory of mind (reasoning about the minds of others of the same species as agents with intentions), and communicating about absent and displaced objects (that have been moved in space or are not present at the time) (CARTA, n.d.).

However, such claims have been contested. Some nonhuman animals have been shown to have many of these capacities, at least in rudimentary form (MacLean, 2016). It is therefore not clear whether humans can be distinguished from other animals on the basis of any single capacity, or even a group of capacities. Perhaps no set of such capacities can provide both necessary and sufficient conditions to distinguish human from nonhuman animals. Moreover, studies claiming to detect these capacities are difficult to carry out and are vigorously debated; many findings may be difficult to replicate; and conceptual frameworks, study methodologies, and interpretations have been debated (Bräuer et al., 2020; Lyn et al., 2014; Tomasello and Call, 2019). Critical literature reviews could help clarify the weight of the current evidence regarding whether animals have specific capacities, and to what degree. Of note, high-level intellectual and cultural achievements, such as proving mathematical theorems, building computers, writing books, and composing operas, are unique to human beings, but are of little help in assessing higher functions in neural organoids and chimeric animals.

Taken together, these considerations suggest that the most informative tests or observations may be those that can show some difference between chimeric and nonchimeric animals of the same species, rather than those that attempt to find "human-like" capacities in a nonhuman animal. These capacities can be assessed by a variety of formal tests described in Chapter 2. In addition, such responses as pain, distress, decreased activity, and social withdrawal can be observed by research veterinarians and animal keepers.[6] If any signs of distress are observed, changes in housing, social environment, activities, and medications can be used to relieve them.

In addition to the above steps, researchers must justify any prospect of increased experience of pain or distress to the IACUC responsible for overseeing the research. If the animal falls under the scope of federal regulations or funding requirements, investigators have specific responsibilities discussed in Chapter 4. Briefly, the researchers must explain to the IACUC how the benefit to human beings of the knowledge gained from the research justifies the pain and distress experienced by the animal as a result of the experiment. Moreover, the IACUC must approve a plan for minimizing and alleviating pain and distress consistent with carrying out the justifiable scientific goals of the research. Although one philosopher suggested that enhanced consciousness would be particularly important ethically if a chimeric animal remembered or anticipated the pain and distress (Piotrowska, 2020), these capacities are not exclusively human or even mammalian characteristics.

---

[6] Megan Albertelli, Stanford University, presentation to the committee, August 11, 2020, virtual meeting. Margaret Landi, GlaxoSmithKline, presentation to the committee, October 30, 2020, virtual meeting.

At present, the issue of altered capacities in chimeric animals is addressed by modifying their care so that pain or suffering is alleviated. In the long term, however, it is possible that a human neural chimera might develop altered capacities, such as those enumerated in Chapter 2, so resembling those of humans that some people might believe such research should not be carried out or that animals of that species should no longer be used in such research, even if the chimera remains a nonhuman animal (Streiffer, 2019). As noted above, others may object to creating any entity that has altered or enhanced capacities, or perhaps even the potential to develop such capacities. A precautionary approach might be warranted, in which enhanced oversight would be introduced at an earlier stage. For example, the field might proceed carefully by pausing when researchers identify changes that differ from species-typical behavior to consider whether those changes are qualitatively different or only small enhancements and whether they have ethical significance. This reflection might be carried out, for example, through bodies that review and oversee such research.

It should be kept in mind that human beings already create nonhuman animals with altered capacities, such as resistance to disease; increased size or speed; or enhanced production of milk, eggs, or wool, In some cases, the selected characteristics are behavioral and therefore likely affect the brain—for example, breeding dogs to have particular skills or greater docility. These modifications have generally been accomplished through selective breeding, but are now beginning to be made by genome modification. Selective breeding at least is widely accepted as falling within responsible human stewardship over nonhuman animals. Generating novel mental capacities in neural transplants and chimeras resembles this type of stewardship in some superficial respects, but differs in the methods used, the involvement of human cells, and the explicit focus on the brain.

Concerns Related to the Use of Nonhuman Primates

Although most neural cell transplants and chimeras currently use rats and mice as the host species, it is likely that some future studies will use nonhuman primates for this purpose. As discussed in Chapter 2, such research holds promise in two respects: Monkeys are likely to be more successful hosts than rodents for generating human neural chimeras or transplants and chimeras are likely to be better models of human brain diseases when the host is a primate rather than a rodent. However, the evolutionary proximity of nonhuman primates to humans that constitutes a scientific advantage also heightens moral and ethical concerns (Feng et al., 2020; Greely, 2021). For example, symptoms of psychiatric disorders, including sadness, decreased interest in activities, disordered sleep, and social isolation, will be more recognizable in nonhuman primates as distinct from species-typical behaviors, but also may be difficult for researchers and veterinarians to ameliorate, as required by animal welfare regulations and ethics. Should they develop, moreover, such enhanced capacities as enhanced problem solving, memory, and self-awareness may appear to be more similar to those of humans in nonhuman primates than in small animals, and may be seen as violating human dignity. Such chimeras could also evoke the specter of more human-like intermediate animals, heightening concerns about the blurring of boundaries between species. For related reasons, animal welfare regulations are already more stringent for nonhuman primates than for rodents, and it is likely that there will be pressure from many quarters to increase this differential for human neural cell transplants and chimeras generated in primate hosts.

Regulatory issues specific to nonhuman primates are detailed in Chapter 4.

ETHICAL ISSUES SPECIFIC TO HUMAN NEURAL ORGANOIDS

This chapter has enumerated a wide range of concerns related to human neural organoid, transplant, and chimera research, as well as concerns specific to transplants and chimeras. Are there concerns specific to neural organoids? In fact, the committee heard about very few ethical concerns regarding current and near-term neural organoid research other than those detailed above.

Because there are no animal hosts, there are no animal welfare concerns and no violations of the foundational cultural distinction between humans and nonhuman animals. Indeed, if the use of human neural organoids can decrease the use of animals in research, that would represent an ethical benefit under the Three R's framework for animal welfare. None of the religious scholars who spoke to the committee or whose work the committee consulted suggest that human neural organoids in vitro would ever acquire the moral status of a human being, undermine the special status of human beings, or otherwise raise theological concerns because in their view, the mere presence of human cells would never make an organoid human.

However, some express revulsion at the possibility that cells taken from their bodies could be used to generate organoids or that brain organoids might develop "human-type awareness" (Smith, 2020). More information is needed to determine whether such responses might be common. For the moment, some of these concerns are alleviated by the fact that, as discussed in Chapter 2, human neural organoids are currently very limited in size, complexity, and maturity and are likely to remain so. They do not meet any current criteria for consciousness and awareness. In the future, however, the complexity of organoids and the circuits they contain will surely increase. It will therefore be essential to revisit these questions as models improve and as understanding of consciousness and awareness changes.

Bioethical analysis could begin by identifying features or capacities that signify moral status and might therefore lead to restrictions on certain types of research. One concern might be that an organoid comprised of human cells achieves consciousness and can experience pain or distress. Aach and colleagues (2017) have discussed ways of considering concerns related to "synthetic human entities with embryo-like features" (SHEEFs), which are not organoids, but the discussion is highly relevant. The authors emphasize the importance of paying attention to concerns that bother people, calling for consideration of "features that directly trigger moral concern..." through "a multi-tracked exploratory inquiry process that both solicits opinions on how SHEEFs might be morally concerning from a wide range of disciplines, traditions, and institutions..." (p. 3 and p. 15). This approach bears some similarity to the consideration of repugnance (the yuck factor) described above. In this inquiry, it will be essential to "identify the biological substrates" of these morally important features or capacities—for example, the neural organization, circuits, and functions that together would be necessary for them to develop—and then "threshold levels for these features and functions that must not be allowed to appear jointly" in a neural organoid or chimera. Thresholds should allow "safety margins to be built into the limits against the possibility of generating" organoids with morally concerning features.

At the level of science policy, if there is broad agreement on features or capacities that raise moral concern and the neural substrates jointly required to achieve them, oversight policies based on avoiding these neural substrates could be crafted. The history of policy debates regarding other technologies, such as genetically modified foods (Scott et al., 2018) and wastewater recycling (Miller, 2012), suggests the value of engaging with the public, understanding and addressing their concerns, and linking research to important unmet needs—for example, unmet needs for treatments for brain diseases—that all can recognize (Lassen, 2018).

SUMMARY

This chapter has reviewed a number of important ethical issues regarding human neural organoid, transplantation, and chimera research. First, there are strong ethical reasons for working to relieve serious human suffering caused by neurological and psychiatric diseases for which effective treatments are lacking or limited (Parker, 2020). Second, there may be concerns about human beings encroaching on divine roles or overreaching appropriate human activities. Third, there may be ethical issues involved in carrying out such research using cells derived from biological materials of persons who did not know their materials were being used for such research and, had they been told, would have objected. Such concerns may be particularly salient in groups that have suffered health disparities and discrimination. Fourth, there are various concerns related to the distinctions between human beings and other animals. Fifth, there are concerns about animal welfare and animal rights. Sixth, there are concerns about consciousness and enhanced capacities in research animals or neural organoids. Finally, there are concerns about the use of nonhuman primates in such research. The committee emphasizes that there are a range of positions on these issues, and that many important issues require discussion among people with different perspectives.

4

Oversight and Governance

The generation of and research on human neural organoids, transplants, and chimeras are subject to a wide range of oversight mechanisms regarding the use of human tissues and stem cells, as well as the use and welfare of nonhuman animals.[1] In the United States, some of this oversight is mandated by federal law, although research may also be subject to state laws and, when it involves collaborating internationally, to regulations in other countries. These legal requirements are often implemented by committees at individual research institutions. There are also de facto limits on research based on what the government or private funders will or will not fund. This collection of laws and regulations is supplemented by nonbinding consensus studies by scientific academies; professional society guidelines; and conference reports by the scientific, bioethics, and advocacy communities. Each of these oversight mechanisms was established to address a specific perceived need within the research enterprise (e.g., protection of human subjects or animal welfare). In contrast, there are few mechanisms for holistic evaluations of new fields of research. This chapter summarizes this patchwork of oversight, including frameworks in other countries. It ends with a review of suggestions that have been made for improving oversight in the future.

A particular challenge to government regulation and voluntary guidelines on research involving human neural organoids, transplants, and chimeras is the broad range of strongly held, and often inconsistent, views in the United States and internationally. Some views are based on religious commitments to different faith traditions, while others are based on secular arguments. Religious commit-

---

[1] Additional rules and guidelines may apply if the research involves human embryos, transgenic animals, pathogens or toxins, certain drugs, or other categories of research.

ments and beliefs are a core source of personal morality and inspiration for many. However, because the United States is a pluralist society, no specific religious tradition may determine public policy. On the other hand, the U.S. National Bioethics Advisory Commission states in its report on cloning of human beings, another deeply contested issue: "Although in a pluralistic society particular religious views cannot be determinative for public policy decisions that bind everyone, policy makers should understand and show respect for diverse moral ideas."[2] Later in this report, this committee articulates the value of ongoing forums for discussion of controversial issues in biotechnology among persons representing different perspectives.

USE OF HUMAN STEM CELLS

Important protections for research participants are provided by the Federal Policy for the Protection of Human Subjects,[3] with oversight by institutional review boards (IRBs) at the respective research institutions. This policy regulates research funded by 18 federal departments and agencies, including the National Institutes of Health (NIH). Part A of this federal policy, known as the Common Rule, was last updated in 2017.[4] Protections mandated by the Common Rule apply when research entails an intervention in or interaction with a living individual or uses identifiable information or biospecimens. Thus, work with tissues and cells from the deceased is not subject to the Common Rule, although other rules (e.g., special funding or review requirements related to embryonic stem cell lines) may apply. Also not subject to the Common Rule is research on existing tissue and cells (for example, from a bank or other collection) for which the living donor's identity is no longer readily ascertainable.

The Common Rule does not apply to all human subjects research done in the United States—research that is done without funding from one of the signatory agencies and that will not be submitted to the Food and Drug Administration (FDA), for example, may not be within its scope, but it is the broadest regulation of such research in the United States and may often provide a framework for oversight of even noncovered work. This is particularly true of major research universities, which may follow the substantive and procedural aspects of the Common Rule for all human subjects research regardless of funding source. The FDA

---

[2] U.S. National Bioethics Advisory Commission, "Cloning Human Beings, Volume 1: Report and Recommendations of the National Bioethics Advisory Commission," 1997, p. 7.

[3] Statutory authority for the regulations for the protection of human subjects derives from the National Research Act of 1974.

[4] 82 Fed. Reg. 12 (January 19, 2017).

has adopted regulations close to but not exactly following the Common Rule on some aspects of consent and consent waivers.[5]

Researchers usually employ stem cells to generate the neural and glial cells used to create human neural organoids, transplants, and chimeras. These stem cells include induced pluripotent stem cells (iPSCs), derived from somatic cells (usually skin or blood cells) of adult donors; embryonic stem cells (ESCs); and, less commonly, fetal cells.[6] Because ESCs raise more ethical, legal, and funding concerns than iPSCs (and entail additional oversight and funding restrictions), researchers often use iPSCs if feasible. Table 4-1 summarizes regulations and guidance on the use of human stem cells for this research.

The Common Rule is heavily influenced by the 1979 Belmont Report of the National Commission for the Protection of Human Subjects of Biomedical and Behavioral Research,[7] as well as, in part, by the Helsinki Declaration, which lays out ethical principles for medical research involving human subjects.[8] Although there are a wide range of policies throughout the world (HHS, 2020), protections for human subjects are broadly recognized.

The Common Rule generally requires IRB approval of human subjects research and contains specific requirements for IRB membership, function, operations, and review of research. The IRB must determine that the research protocol meets specified criteria, including reasonable risks in relation to anticipated benefits, equitable subject selection, protection of confidentiality of the research participants, adequate informed consent, and participant safety. The focus for IRBs in overseeing research on human neural organoids and transplants (and potential future research involving chimeras) is on obtaining informed consent for donation of human biospecimens; protecting the privacy interests of living, identifiable donors; and, if donors placed special limits on the use of their cells, ensuring research use consistent with those limits.

Transplantation of human neural cells or organoids into humans would be subject to both additional oversight by IRBs (because the human transplant recipient would also be a human subject) and additional review by the FDA pursuant to its authorities that cover granting permission to begin clinical trials or marketing of human cell, tissue, and cellular- and tissue-based products.[9]

At many institutions, research using human ESCs or iPSCs is subject to additional oversight by Embryonic Stem Cell Research Oversight (ESCRO) commit-

---

[5] If or when organoids or human cells are transplanted into animals that are used for therapeutic purposes, any research that supports a commercial product application to the FDA will also need to comply with FDA regulations for protection of human subjects (21 C.F.R. 50).

[6] Research involving fetal tissues is subject to a wide range of rules and oversight, which were summarized for the committee by Valerie Bonham and Mark Barnes, Ropes & Gray LLP, at its November 13, 2020, virtual meeting, are not discussed in more detail in this chapter.

[7] See https://www.hhs.gov/ohrp/regulations-and-policy/belmont-report/read-the-belmont-report/index.html.

[8] The Declaration of Helsinki was last revised in 2013 (World Medical Association, 1964).

[9] 21 C.F.R. § 1271.

TABLE 4-1 Oversight of Research Based on the Use of Human Stem Cells

Type of Research	Common Rule (federal regulations for research funded by U.S. government)	National Institutes of Health (NIH) Guidelines for Human Stem Cell Research (funding requirement)	Nonbinding Guidance
Research using human induced pluripotent stem cells (iPSCs) from deidentified donor cells (e.g., from a biobank)	Exempt from institutional review boards (IRB) review if cells are appropriately deidentified	N/A	Exempt from Embryonic Stem Cell Research Oversight (ESCRO) committee review (NRC and IOM, 2010) Exempt from Embryonic Research Oversight (EMRO) review (ISSCR, 2016)
Research using human iPSCs from identifiable donor cells	IRB oversight to determine appropriate informed consent (including broad consent or waiver of consent), confidentiality, etc.	N/A	IRB review should determine that informed consent includes the possibility of use in animals (NRC and IOM, 2010, ISSCR, 2016)
Research using deidentified human embryonic stem cells (ESCs) (e.g., from a biobank)	Exempt from IRB review if cells are appropriately deidentified	Specific requirements for origin of cells, including consent from donors of embryos and gametes	ESCRO should determine that cells were "acceptably derived" (NRC and IOM, 2010) No specialized EMRO review (ISSCR, 2016)
Research using identifiable human ESCs	IRB oversight to determine appropriate informed consent, confidentiality, etc.	Specific requirements for origin of cells, including consent from donors of embryos and gametes	Review by ESCRO (NRC and IOM, 2010) Review by EMRO (ISSCR, 2016)

NOTE: Additional oversight is required if the use of human stem cells includes transplantation into a nonhuman animal (see Table 4-2).

tees or Stem Cell Research Oversight (SCRO) committees, which are generally described in the National Academies Guidelines for Human Embryonic Stem Cell Research, first published in 2005 and most recently updated in 2010 (NRC and IOM, 2010). These committees ensure that the research follows federal, state, and funding agency guidelines and has undergone appropriate scientific and ethical review. The National Academies guidelines provide recommendations on the membership of ESCROs, which should include individuals with expertise in developmental biology, stem cell research, molecular biology, assisted reproduction, and ethical and legal issues in human embryonic stem cell research. A nonscientist member of the public not affiliated with the institution should also be included. The International Society for Stem Cell Research (ISSCR) Guidelines for Stem Cell Research and Clinical Translation (2016; update expected in 2021) recommend a similar type of oversight (ISSCR, 2016).

Although the guidelines of the National Academies and the ISSCR are nonbinding, both are widely followed by institutions that conduct this type of research. Some states, including California[10] and New York (Shah, 2013), have made oversight by an ESCRO or SCRO committee mandatory for research funded by the state. ESCROs, SCROs, or Embryonic Research Oversight (EMRO) committees could consider a wide range of ethical issues related to research involving human stem cells, including the possibility of altered capacities in chimeric animals or the development of consciousness in organoids, but there is very little information about how these committees function at different institutions.

In general, guidance related to the disposal of human tissue from liveborn human beings that is used in research is designed to protect researchers, clinicians, and others from harms that might arise from those tissues, such as infectious diseases or environmental contamination. Some organizations providing tissue may specify requirements for disposal or return of unused material through material transfer agreements, but this is negotiated between the parties. The Common Rule, National Academies guidelines, and ISSCR guidelines do not address disposal, indicating that such issues have not generally been seen as raising ethical concerns. In practice, in research laboratories, disposal of human neural tissues does not differ from disposal of other biomaterials.

INFORMED CONSENT

Ethical issues surrounding informed consent are discussed in Chapter 3; the oversight mechanisms described here were established to address many of those concerns, although it is important to remember that the legal regulation around informed consent may not be coextensive with those ethical issues. Informed consent is a key requirement of the Common Rule, which requires investigators to provide prospective research subjects the information necessary for them to make an informed and voluntary decision about whether to participate in the research.[11] The requirements for consent from participants for an initial donation of tissues (e.g., skin cells that will be used to generate iPSCs) differ from those for use of existing biospecimens in subsequent studies.

---

[10] California Institute of Regenerative Medicine Regulations § 10060 (SCRO Committee Membership and Function) and § 10070 (SCRO Committee Review and Notification).

[11] 45 C.F.R. § 46.116.

Collection of New Biospecimens for Research

New biospecimens may be collected for research in two ways. First, if biospecimens are obtained specifically for research, informed consent is required from the donor. Ethically, researchers must disclose information that reasonable people would want to know about how their tissues will be used. Many might argue that this information should include any intention at the time of collection to use the tissues to generate a neural organoid or to transplant derived materials into a nonhuman animal. However, this is not required in current regulations, and IRBs can differ in how they interpret what a "reasonable" person might want to know before donating. The regulations require that participants be informed that deidentified biospecimens and information might be used for future research or shared with other investigators without additional consent. When applicable, research participants must be informed of possible commercial profit from the research (and whether they will share in this profit), whether research activities will or might include whole genetic sequencing, and whether clinically relevant research results will be returned to participants. As of 2015, NIH funding policy for genomic studies requires "explicit consent for participants' genomic and phenotypic data (which may include some clinical information) to be used for future research purposes and to be shared broadly through data repositories" (NIH, 2019).

A second approach to obtaining new biospecimens for research is to derive them from tissue or cells considered surgical or medical waste. If these specimens are collected and used in a manner such that the identity of the people from whom they were derived cannot be readily ascertained by the researchers, the activity is not considered human subjects research, and consent is not required. If identifying links are retained, consent is necessary as described above.

Obtaining consent to use biospecimens and data for future research is challenging because it is impossible to anticipate or describe all future research projects. The 2017 revisions to the Common Rule allow biospecimens or information to be used in future research or shared with other researchers—for example, through a biobank—without additional consent.

The most commonly used approach to obtaining consent for future research and sharing of biospecimens and information with other researchers is deidentification: donors are told that future research and sharing might be carried out in such a way that "the identity of the human subjects cannot readily be ascertained directly or through identifiers linked to the subjects, the investigator does not contact the subjects, and the investigator will not re-identify subjects."[12] In everyday discussions, the literature, and this report, such specimens are called "deidentified," and the persons who provide the materials for research are called "donors." With such disclosure, future research and sharing are permitted without additional consent.

An alternative to obtaining consent for future research and sharing of *identifiable* specimens and information is broad consent. The research subject must be

---

[12] 45 C.F.R. § 46.104 (d)(4)(ii).

given a general description of the types of research that may be conducted, in sufficient detail that a "reasonable person would expect that the broad consent would permit the types of research conducted."[13] For broad consent, donors must be told that they will not be informed of the details of such specific research studies and that they might have chosen not to consent to some of those specific research studies.[14]

Research with Existing Biospecimens

As discussed above, secondary research with deidentified existing biospecimens and data is not considered human subjects research, and additional consent or full IRB review is not required. This policy lies at the heart of some of the ethical concerns with tissue- and cell-based research. While a person who is unidentifiable may have no privacy interests to protect, that person may nonetheless be unhappy at having unwittingly contributed to a form or research that he or she views as immoral or emotionally disturbing. This is one example in which the regulatory protections do not extend as far as what some would argue are legitimate ethical concerns, although extending the regulations to such situations would arguably undermine other values, such as the interest in health-promoting scientific research.

To protect the identity of the donors, a biobank can share specimens together with associated phenotypic information after replacing personal identifiers with a code number that is not shared with the secondary researchers. In one approach to deidentification, the biobank destroys the links between the code numbers and overt identifiers. In another approach, the biobank retains the links but adopts a policy of never sharing them with secondary researchers. Of note, deidentifying specimens and data precludes recontacting donors—for example, to inform them of clinically actionable research findings. Providing deidentified specimens and data simplifies the oversight process for secondary researchers. However, there are growing concerns, discussed below, about the ability of new technologies to "reidentify" donors of nominally "deidentified" tissue.

In addition to situations that involve carrying out future research and sharing deidentified specimens, additional consent and full IRB review are not required in two other cases. First, as discussed previously, if biospecimens and information remain identifiable but were collected with broad consent for future research, the additional research may proceed without additional consent if the IRB ascertains that the proposed new research falls within the terms of original donation of the biospecimens. Second, for other research using existing identified biospecimens or information, secondary researchers may request a waiver or alteration of informed consent under certain circumstances.

---

[13] 45 C.F.R. § 46.116(d).
[14] 45 C.F.R. § 46.116(d).

USE AND CARE OF ANIMALS IN RESEARCH

Research involving human neural cell transplants into nonhuman animals or chimeras is subject to the rules and regulations related to the use of animals in research, including oversight by institutional animal care and use committees (IACUCs), which are mandated at the federal level. The Animal Welfare Act (AWA) of 1966 is overseen by the U.S. Department of Agriculture's (USDA's) Animal and Plant Health Inspection Service and applies to all research on warm-blooded animals (excluding birds, rats, and mice raised for the purpose of laboratory use), regardless of the source of funding.[15] In addition, the Public Health Service Policy on Humane Care and Use of Laboratory Animals (PHS Policy), last updated in 2015, covers all live vertebrate animals involved in activities funded by agencies within the PHS, including NIH, the FDA, and the Centers for Disease Control and Prevention (CDC).[16] The PHS Policy incorporates the 1985 U.S. Government Principles for the Utilization and Care of Vertebrate Animals Used in Testing, Research and Training (U.S. Government Principles) (NIH, 2018), which apply to all federal agencies. The PHS Policy and the U.S. Government Principles help define best practices for animal use and care and are widely followed even by institutions that do not receive federal funding. The PHS Policy has also adopted guidance developed by the National Academies (Guide for the Care and Use of Laboratory Animals, last updated in 2011 [NRC, 2011]) and the American Veterinary Medical Association (Guidelines on Euthanasia of Animals, last updated in 2020 [AVMA, 2020]). IACUCs ensure compliance with this range of government laws, policies, and guidance.

Federal regulations require that research protocols describe the research, approaches used to reduce animal numbers, justification for the use of animals, information on alleviation of pain and distress, methods of euthanasia, an understanding of the scientific literature, and plans for appropriate veterinary care. The committee notes that the requirement to justify the use of animals in terms of prospective benefit to human health in the case of neural cell transplant and chimera research goes conceptually beyond the Three R's framework (*r*educe, *r*efine, and *r*eplace) described in Chapter 3. These protocols must be reviewed and approved by an IACUC, with periodic review of ongoing research. According to the PHS Policy, IACUCs must have a minimum of five members, including one doctor of veterinary medicine with training or experience in laboratory animal science and medicine who has direct or delegated program authority and responsibilities for activities involving the animals at the institution, one practicing scientist experienced in research involving animals, one member whose primary concerns are in a nonscientific area (e.g., an ethicist, lawyer, or member of the clergy), and one individual who is not affiliated with the institution in any way other than as

---

[15] 7 U.S.C. §§ 2131–2159 (Pub. L. 89-544), with implementing regulations: 9 C.F.R., § 1(A).

[16] See https://olaw.nih.gov/policies-laws/phs-policy.htm. Statutory authority derives from the Health Research Extension Act of 1985, 42 U.S.C. Ch. 6A(II)(A), (III, § 283[e]), and (III, Part H, §289d), Pub. L. 99-158 (11/20/85).

a member of the IACUC and has no immediate family members affiliated with the institution.

Under the PHS Policy and U.S. Government Principles, proper use of research animals includes avoidance and minimization of discomfort, distress, and pain, as well as due consideration of the potential benefits of the research. Unless the contrary is established, procedures that cause pain in humans are assumed to cause pain in nonhuman animals.[17] Procedures that cause more than momentary or slight pain or distress must be performed with appropriate sedation, analgesics, or anesthetics unless withholding of such agents is justified for scientific reasons and approved by the IACUC. Animals that would experience severe or chronic pain or distress that cannot be relieved must be painlessly euthanized at the end of the procedure, or if appropriate, during the procedure. No animal should be used in more than one major operative procedure from which it is allowed to recover unless justified for scientific reasons.

Both the National Academies Guide for the Care and Use of Laboratory Animals (NRC, 2011) and the American Veterinary Medical Association's Guidelines for Euthanasia of Animals (AMVA, 2020) provide guidance on the disposal of nonhuman animal remains once an experiment has been completed. Both sets of guidelines focus on protecting the environment and other animals from infectious diseases or chemical contaminants, and indicate no differential considerations based on the characteristics of the animal. Researchers working with animals with human neural cell transplants or chimeric animals would follow these same guidelines.

The principles that underlie the U.S. approach to oversight of animal research are broadly accepted. The Association for Assessment and Accreditation of Laboratory Animal Care International (AAALAC International), a nonprofit organization that promotes the humane treatment of animals in science through voluntary accreditation and assessment programs, has accredited research facilities in 49 countries.[18] Directive 2010/63/EU in the European Union includes the Three R's and requires institutional oversight bodies similar to IACUCs.[19] Both the EU Directive and AAALAC accreditation require protections for cephalopods in addition to vertebrate animals. China, Japan, and Singapore have also adopted guidelines to ensure appropriate oversight for the use and care of animals in research (NRC, 2012). Japan's Act on Welfare and Management of Animals, most recently amended in 2014, explicitly incorporates the Three R's principles.[20]

---

[17] NRC, 2011 (see Appendix B: U.S. Government Principles for the Utilization and Care of Vertebrate Animals Used in Testing, Research and Training, Principle IV); CIMS and ICLAS, 2012 (see Principle VII).

[18] AAALAC accreditation standards include adherence to the National Academies' *Guide to the Care and Use of Laboratory Animals* (NRC, 2011), which are also adopted by the U.S. PHS Policy.

[19] Directive 2010/63/EU of the European Parliament and of the Council of 22 September 2010 on the protection of animals used for scientific purposes. See https://eur-lex.europa.eu/legal-content/EN/TXT/?uri=CELEX:32010L0063.

[20] Act on Welfare and Management of Animals (Act. No. 105 of October 1, 1973, as amended by Act No. 46 of May 30, 2014). See http://www.env.go.jp/nature/dobutsu/aigo/1_law/files/aigo_kanri_1973_105_en.pdf.

China in 2016 adopted its first national standards governing the treatment of laboratory animals, which cover euthanasia, pain management, transport and housing; breeding facilities; and personnel training (McLaughlin, 2016).

USE OF NONHUMAN PRIMATES IN RESEARCH

The use of nonhuman primates raises obligations that go beyond those required for other research animals. The AWA includes provisions to ensure the psychological well-being of nonhuman primates,[21] including, at a minimum, addressing their social needs and social groupings, providing adequate environmental enrichment, and not maintaining them in restraint devices for longer than required to attain the approved scientific goals of the research or for more than 12 hours continuously. The AWA regulations require certain nonhuman primates to be provided special attention regarding enhancement of their environment, based on the needs of the individual species and in accordance with the instructions of the attending veterinarian. Nonhuman primates requiring special attention include infants and young juveniles; those that show signs of being in psychological distress through behavior or appearance; those used in research for which the committee-approved protocol requires restricted activity; individually housed nonhuman primates that are unable to see and hear nonhuman primates of their own or compatible species; and great apes weighing more than 110 lb.[22] USDA conducts inspections of U.S. research institutions that conduct research on nonhuman primates to ensure compliance with the AWA. Institutions that conduct research on chimpanzees and other great apes take extra precautions to ensure compliance both to fulfill their ethical obligations to the animals and to meet the high expectations of the public.

In the United States, the use of nonhuman primates in research has received scrutiny in recent years, including legislation to limit the use of these animals.[23] In December 2010, NIH commissioned a study by the Institute of Medicine (IOM) to assess whether and to what extent chimpanzees are necessary and will be necessary in the future for biomedical and behavioral research. The IOM issued its findings in 2011, with a primary recommendation that the use of chimpanzees in research be guided by a set of principles including (1) that the knowledge gained must be necessary to advance the public's health; (2) that there must be no other research model by which the knowledge could be obtained, and the research cannot be ethically performed on human subjects; and (3) that the animals used in the proposed research be maintained either in ethologically appropriate physical and social environments or in natural habitats (IOM, 2011). The report concludes that chimpanzee research has been a valuable research animal model but that most

---

[21] Animal Welfare Act (7 U.S.C. § 2143).
[22] 9 C.F.R., Ch. 1(A), Animal Welfare, Part 3, § 3.81(c).
[23] The Further Consolidated Appropriations Act, 2020 (Pub. L. 116-94, December 20, 2019) requires special authorization by the Secretary of Veterans Affairs for that agency's research use of nonhuman primates, felines, or canines; requires NIH to explore alternatives to the use of nonhuman primates; and requires the FDA to develop a detailed plan for reduction and retirement of its monkeys.

current uses of chimpanzees for biomedical research are unnecessary. Later, a working group convened by an NIH advisory body evaluated specific experiments and went into more depth on the enhanced living conditions (CCWG, 2013). NIH subsequently announced plans to phase out much of the research that involves these animals (NIH, 2013) and no longer funds biomedical research on chimpanzees (Collins, 2015). NIH has continued efforts to improve the rigor and reproducibility of research involving nonhuman primates more broadly—for example, with a workshop on the topic in February 2020 (AAMC, 2020). Of note, privately funded research may continue and is not subject to the limitations and conditions recommended by the IOM and the NIH working group.

Animal welfare laws in many other countries are more restrictive than those in the United States regarding the use of nonhuman primates. Under the Directive 2010/63/EU, biomedical research on nonhuman primates is allowed only when no alternatives are available for basic research, when it is focused on preservation of the primate species, or when the work addresses potentially life-threatening or debilitating conditions in humans. Research involving chimpanzees and other great apes is allowed in very rare circumstances. The United Kingdom, Germany, the Netherlands, Sweden, Austria,[24] Belgium, Japan, and New Zealand[25] go further than the EU Directive and have policies or laws that essentially ban the use of great apes (but not monkeys) as laboratory animals (Knight, 2008; Should apes have legal rights, 2013). In these jurisdictions, a researcher seeking to transplant human cells into a nonhuman primate would face significant hurdles.

U.S. POLICY AND GUIDANCE SPECIFIC TO NEURAL TRANSPLANTS AND CHIMERAS

Table 4-2 summarizes U.S. laws, policies, and nonbinding guidance covering neural cell transplants and human neural chimeras. Beyond the provisions of the AWA and PHS Policy addressing research animals, there are no provisions in U.S. federal law specific to the generation of human-animal chimeras or to ensuring their welfare and well-being (although two U.S. states have laws barring the creation of some human neural chimeras[26]). In recent years, however, the use of human stem cells for neural cell transplants into nonhuman animals or for generation of human neural chimeras has been the subject of policy discussions at NIH. The

---

[24] Austria's Animal Experiments Act of 2012 prohibits animal experiments on the great apes and gibbons.

[25] New Zealand's Animal Welfare Act of 1999 restricts research involving the use of nonhuman hominids to research in the best interest of the species. See http://legislation.govt.nz/act/public/1999/0142/latest/DLM51206.html.

[26] Arizona and Louisiana prohibit the generation of a "human-animal hybrid," which is defined in part as a nonhuman life form engineered so that it contains a human brain or a brain derived "wholly or predominantly" from human neural tissue. The Louisiana law also includes a clause barring the creation of a nonhuman embryo into which human cells or cell components have been introduced (Louisiana Revised Statutes §14:89.6.A [2018]; Arizona Revised Statutes Ann § 36-2311 [2013]). See also Macintosh (2015).

TABLE 4-2 Oversight Specific to Human Neural Cell Transplants and Neural Chimeras

Procedure	Animal Use and Welfare Laws in the United States	National Institutes of Health (NIH) Guidelines and Policy Development (funding requirements)
Neural cell transplants made by grafting human cells into a fetal or postnatal nonprimate vertebrate (e.g., mouse) brain	Review by institutional animal care and use committees (IACUC)	Proposal for additional oversight of research that shows a "substantial contribution or a substantial functional modification to the animal brain by the human cells"
Neural cell transplant made by grafting human cells into a fetal or postnatal nonhuman primate brain	Review by IACUC, with additional protections and oversight for nonhuman primates, including measures to promote psychological well-being	Proposal for additional oversight of research that shows a "substantial contribution or a substantial functional modification to the animal brain by the human cells"
Chimera made by inserting human cells into a nonprimate vertebrate (e.g., mouse) blastocyst	Review by IACUC Likely forbidden in Arizona and Louisiana	Funding moratorium. Proposal for additional oversight of research that shows a "substantial contribution or a substantial functional modification to the animal brain by the human cells" Breeding is forbidden where human cells may contribute to germline. (NIH Guidelines for Human Stem Cell Research)
Chimera made by inserting human cells into a nonhuman primate blastocyst	Review by IACUC, with additional protections and oversight for nonhuman primates, including measures to promote psychological well-being Forbidden in California; likely forbidden in Arizona and Louisiana.	Forbidden (NIH, 2009)

NOTE: Additional oversight may apply if the human cells are derived from embryonic stem cells (ESCs) rather than induced pluripotent stem cells (iPSCs) or somatic sources (see Table 4-1).

Nonbinding Guidance

Review required, with more careful consideration for fetal transplantation "because the extent of human contribution the resulting animal may be higher" (NRC and IOM, 2010)

Specialized review when the degree of functional integration into the central nervous system may substantially alter the animal host; best practices for ensuring animal welfare (ISSCR, 2016)

Review required, with more careful consideration for fetal transplantation "because the extent of human contribution to the resulting animal may be higher" (NRC and IOM, 2010)

Specialized review when the degree of functional integration into the central nervous system may substantially alter the animal host; especially rigorous for nonhuman primates; best practices for ensuring animal welfare (ISSCR, 2016)

Additional review, with particular attention to the level of functional integration of human cells into the animal; should be considered only under circumstances in which no other experiment can provide the information needed; breeding should not be allowed if human cells may contribute to germline (NRC and IOM, 2010)

Specialized review when the degree of functional integration into the central nervous system may substantially alter the animal host or when human cells may contribute to gametes; best practices for ensuring animal welfare (ISSCR, 2016)

This type of research should not be conducted at this time (NRC and IOM, 2010)

Specialized review when the degree of functional integration into the central nervous system may substantially alter the animal host or when human cells may contribute to gametes; especially rigorous for nonhuman primates; best practices for ensuring animal welfare (ISSCR, 2016)

2009 NIH Guidelines for Human Stem Cell Research[27] prohibit NIH from funding research that introduces human pluripotent stem cells (hPSCs) into nonhuman primate blastocysts (the state of California has a similar prohibition for research funded by the state[28]). It also prohibits funding of research that involves breeding of any research animal whereby human stem cells may contribute to its germline.

In 2015, citing potential ethical and animal welfare concerns and in preparation for additional policy making, NIH issued a moratorium on its funding of research that introduces hPSCs into pregastrulation embryos of any nonhuman vertebrate animal.[29] This moratorium still allows neural cell transplants in which human stem cells are introduced into fetal or postnatal animal brains, but prohibits techniques that introduce human stem cells at early embryonic stages, including blastocyst chimerism and complementation, discussed in Chapter 2.

After imposing the moratorium and hosting a workshop on the topic in November 2015 (OSP, 2015), NIH issued a notice of proposed changes to its guidelines to include the establishment of an NIH steering committee that would provide additional oversight for neural cell transplants and human neural chimeras. NIH proposed that this committee could oversee research involving the introduction of human stem cells early in embryonic development in any vertebrate animal, as well as studies (excluding those in mice) in which human stem cells introduced at any developmental stage could result in "a substantial contribution or a substantial functional modification to the animal brain by the human cells" (OSP, 2016). Such a policy would provide additional oversight for neural cell transplants and human neural chimeras of all types. NIH sought public input on the proposed changes in 2016,[30] but they have never been finalized. The moratorium remains in effect.

The 2010 National Academies Guidelines for Human Embryonic Stem Cell Research, adopted in 2005 and last amended in 2010, explicitly use a three-tiered approach (see the further discussion of such an approach in the next section). The guidelines do not permit the injection of human stem cells (derived from embryos or other sources) into nonhuman primate blastocysts or breeding of nonhuman animals in which such cells could potentially contribute to the germline.[31] The guidelines require additional review for research that introduces human ESCs (hESCs) into nonhuman animals at any stage of development. An ESCRO committee should oversee such research that may result in functional integration of the human cells into the animal. The guidelines provide similar oversight for

---

[27] See https://stemcells.nih.gov/policy/2009-guidelines.htm.

[28] California Institute for Regenerative Medicine, CIRM Medical and Ethical Standards Regulations, § 100030(c) (available at https://www.cirm.ca.gov/sites/default/files/files/board_meetings/CIRM_MES_regulations_Full_Revised_07_17_20 13.pdf).

[29] September 23, 2015. Notice Number: NOT-OD-15-158. See https://grants.nih.gov/grants/guide/notice-files/NOT- OD-15-158.html.

[30] 81 Fed. Reg. 51921. Request for Public Comment on the Proposed Changes to the NIH Guidelines for Human Stem Cell Research and the Proposed Scope of an NIH Steering Committee's Consideration of Certain Human-Animal Chimera Research. August 5, 2016.

[31] NRC and IOM, 2010, §§ 1.3(c) and 7.3(iii[2]).

transplantation into nonhuman animals of hPSCs derived from sources other than human embryos, requiring additional ESCRO review for experiments "where there is a significant possibility that the implanted hPS cells could give rise to neural or gametic cells and tissues."[32] For research involving the use of human stem cells in primates or in cases in which human stem cells may give rise to neural tissues in any nonhuman animal, "particular attention should be paid to at least three factors: the extent to which the implanted cells colonize and integrate into the animal tissue; the degree of differentiation of the implanted cells; and the possible effects of the implanted cells on the function of the animal tissue."[33]

The National Academies guidelines, in sections related to the use of hESC lines, make a distinction between grafting of such cells into adult animal brains (which the guidelines consider to require a lower level of review) and grafting them into fetal animal brains, which would require "more careful consideration because the extent of human contribution to the resulting animal may be higher."[34] The guidelines flag these issues for ethical consideration, but do not offer additional guidance for ensuring the welfare or well-being of chimeras or nonhuman animals with neural cell transplants.

The 2016 ISSCR Guidelines for Stem Cell Research and Clinical Translation address research involving transplantation of human cells into nonhuman animal brains or generation of human-animal chimeras. Although these guidelines do not explicitly follow the three-tiered approach described above, they provide similar guidance. They state that research may require specialized review if human cells have the potential for a high degree of integration into an animal's central nervous system or if they may generate human gametes in nonhuman animal hosts. If the research involves nonhuman primates, this review should be "especially rigorous."

The ISSCR guidelines also recommend best practices for ensuring animal welfare if and when "the degree of functional integration of human cells is considerable enough to raise concerns that the nature of the animal host may be significantly altered." These best practices include: "(a) establishment of baseline animal data; (b) ongoing data collection of deviations from the norms of species typical animals; (c) the use of small pilot studies to ascertain welfare changes in modified animals; and (d) ongoing monitoring and reporting to oversight committee authorized to decide if there is need to change protocols or remove animal subjects from research."[35] As of this writing, these guidelines are undergoing review and revision but have not yet been issued.

Box 4-1 presents scenarios illustrating how different committees might oversee research involving human neural organoids or transplants.

---

[32] NRC and IOM, 2010, § 7.3.
[33] NRC and IOM, 2010, §§ 1.3(b[iii]) and 7.3(ii).
[34] NRC and IOM, 2010, §§ 6.5 and 6.6.
[35] ISSCR, 2016, Recommendation 2.1.5.

BOX 4-1
Illustrative Oversight Scenarios

These scenarios illustrate regulatory structures relevant to research involving neural organoids, transplants, and chimeras with two simple case studies.

Scenario 1: Human Neural Organoid

A researcher at an American university wants to generate and analyze human neural organoids. Her goal is to test the usefulness of such organoids for finding neural abnormalities that might play a role in determining the severity of major depressive disorder, with the hope that these could eventually serve as targets for new therapeutic approaches. Because there are no single genes known to "cause" the disorder, it will not be possible to genetically engineer available stem cells. Therefore, the researcher must obtain small tissue samples (skin or blood) from individuals with clinically validated major depression and reprogram cells to generate induced pluripotent stem cells (iPSCs), which can then be used to form organoids. She will also need samples from age-, race- and gender-matched neurotypical individuals.

To conduct any of these experiments in the United States, the researcher's laboratory must comply with institutional, state, and federal laboratory safety regulations. To collect tissue from which iPSCs can be generated, the researcher will need to have her university's institutional review board (IRB) review and approve her protocol for collecting cells, including the process of obtaining informed consent and measures to protect donor confidentiality (such as removing overt identifiers and using codes instead). Confidentiality is particularly important in this case because major depression is a sensitive diagnosis and may be stigmatizing. It is possible that iPSCs have been collected from individuals with depression in the past and stored in a biobank. These could be useful if other studies were conducted on those individuals. To use such cells, however, or to use commonly available fibroblast cell lines, the researcher may need to demonstrate to the IRB that the cells (together with accompanying clinical information) are "deidentified," that is, cannot readily be linked to any individual, and are being used in ways consistent with the original consent from the donor. Deidentification can be carried out using a code, with the researcher having no access to the key that links the code to overt patient identifiers.[a]

Depending on the type of stem cell used to generate the organoids, additional review may be required. Most major American universities have an institutional Embryonic Stem Cell Research Oversight (ESCRO) committee, Stem Cell Research Oversight (SCRO) committee, or an Embryonic Research Oversight (EMRO) process.[b] These entities vary substantially in whether they look only at research involving embryonic stem cells (ESCs) or also consider iPSCs and if so, in which projects—usually those that involve the generation of human gametes that will be fertilized. If the cells, and hence the research, are covered by the relevant committee, it will review the research protocol for certain issues, such as provenance and consented uses of the cells. Within the laboratory, the research will be covered by institutional and, in some cases, federal regulations governing the use of reagents, potentially including biologics, viral vectors, toxins, or radioactive probes.

Notably, at no point under current law will the researcher have to consider the characteristics, treatment, or condition of the organoids. Given current understanding, organoids are neither human subjects nor research animals. The oversight of organoids addresses only the ethical concerns regarding the human donors of the cells from which they are developed.

Scenario 2: Human Neural Cell Transplant into an Animal

A researcher at an American university wants to transplant human neural stem cells derived from patients with early-onset schizophrenia and from neurotypical individuals into the brains of neonatal mice. The research animals will be allowed to develop to maturity, then euthanized, and their brains will be analyzed. The stem cells will be marked with an indelible (genetically encoded) label so they can later be distinguished from host cells. The aim is to determine whether morphological or physiological properties of the neurons derived from the transplanted cells differ depending on whether the donor was schizophrenic or neurotypical. This is regarded as a step in developing a model for this disease.

Regulations governing human subjects, consent, and derivation of iPSCs are identical to those described above for Scenario 1. In this case, review and approval of the protocol by the university's institutional animal care and use committee (IACUC) is also required to ensure the welfare of nonhuman animals in research. The IACUC will review the protocol to ensure that the animals will be treated humanely and that the potential benefits of the research justify the harms to the animals. In addition, the treatment of the animals will be governed and overseen throughout the study by regulations, policies, and practices implemented by the university's laboratory animal group, which will include veterinarians with species-relevant experience. The protocol will need to specify how symptoms of distress will be identified and alleviated. The IACUC will determine whether and to what extent the researcher should consider assessing the animals for altered or unusual capacities.

To assess a protocol that involves neural cell transplantation into an animal, IACUCs need relevant experience with animal models, including those engrafted with human tissues in organs other than brain, and also with a variety of neural transgenic models, including nonhuman primate models of Huntington's disease and autism. To provide appropriate oversight for specific types of research, an IACUC may reach out to IACUCs at other institutions to request outside expertise or appoint subject matter experts to serve as ad hoc members on the committee.

[a]See page 71 of the current report for a more detailed examination of the challenges with deidentification.
[b]As discussed on page 68 of the current report.

GRADED OVERSIGHT: A THREE-TIERED APPROACH

Over the past several years, a three-tiered approach has been proposed for the guidance of research in biotechnological areas that raise substantial ethical and regulatory concerns.

The first tier is research that can be reviewed and approved by existing oversight mechanisms because it presents no new ethical or regulatory concerns beyond those the current oversight system is charged with addressing. Most current research discussed in this report involving human organoids, human neural cell transplants, and chimeras involving nonhuman donors and nonprimate hosts falls into this category.

The second tier is research that can proceed after additional review and approval. Broadly speaking, such research raises additional ethical concerns that the current oversight system, such as IRBs and IACUCs, is not designed to address. The additional review that is required for this tier of research may be carried out through institutional or national committees. Research that falls into this tier might include neural transplants that render the host's brain more "human-like," particularly in nonhuman primates.

The third tier is research that should not be permitted at the present time. This category includes experiments that are currently forbidden under U.S. law, including the introduction of hESCs or iPSCs into the blastocyst of a nonhuman animal.

Several National Academies committees have recommended a three-tiered oversight structure for other types of innovative biomedical research—for example, human genome editing (NASEM, 2017a, pp. 181–194). Several other countries have also adopted this approach, as described in the next section, which includes an expanded description of policies in the United Kingdom.

Table 4-3 provides examples of experiments involving human neural organoids, transplants, or chimeras that fall into each of these tiers under the current U.S. regulatory framework: (1) research that can proceed under existing oversight mechanisms, (2) research that may require additional review, and (3) research that should not proceed at this time.

INTERNATIONAL POLICY SPECIFIC TO NEURAL ORGANOIDS, TRANSPLANTS, AND CHIMERAS

The committee could find no laws, policies, or guidance at the national level in any country addressing the creation of human neural organoids beyond those focused on broad categories of in vitro research that might include such organoids. However, several countries have policies that include provisions for the transplantation of human stem cells into nonhuman animals, and these policies show a range of approaches. The ISSCR guidelines, described above, are influential in much of the world and provide additional relevant guidance for scientists and institutions. Laws that provide protections for animals used in research are

TABLE 4-3 Examples of Human Neural Organoid, Transplant, and Chimera Research Subject to Different Levels of Scrutiny

Green Level of Scrutiny: Research That Can Proceed Under Existing Oversight Mechanisms

Neural Organoids	Neural Cell Transplants	Neural Chimeras
Generation of human neural organoids from human patient-derived iPSCs for use to understand human brain formation, identify disease-related abnormalities, and screen drugs that reverse those abnormalities	Transplantation of human ESC- or iPSC-derived neural progenitors into the nervous system of wild-type mice and mice that model brain disease to assess whether the milieu affects their differentiation, connections, and function	Generation of chimeras in which human ESCs or iPSCs are implanted into the blastocyst of a nonhuman animal and maintained solely in vitro

Yellow Level of Scrutiny: Research That May Require Additional Review

Neural Organoids	Neural Cell Transplants	Neural Chimeras
Experiments using iPSCs to generate neural organoids when there is ambiguity about the human donor's consent.	Transplantation of large numbers of human ESC- or iPSC-derived neural progenitors into the cortex of a neonatal macaque such that integration into circuits might lead to altered behavior	Transplantation of human cells into mouse blastocysts followed by implantation into the uterus of a host mouse.

Red Level of Scrutiny: Research That Should Not Proceed at This Time

Neural Organoids	Neural Cell Transplants	Neural Chimeras
Experiments using iPSCs to generate neural organoids that violate the terms of the human donor's consent	Studies where human stem cells introduced into nonhuman primate embryos with the aim of populating the developing neural tube could result in generation of donor-derived gametes in the host	Transplantation of human cells into blastocysts of nonhuman primates followed by implantation into the uterus of a host

common in the developed world, as discussed above, and add another layer of oversight for this type of research.

Several countries have developed official policy or guidance on the transfer of human cells into nonhuman animals that follows the three-tiered approach to oversight described in the preceding section, identifying research that can proceed under existing oversight mechanisms; research that may require additional review; and research that should be prohibited.

In 2011, the German National Ethics Council issued additional guidance applying the Embryo Protection Act of 1990 to address newer laboratory techniques, including the possibility of using human iPSCs in human neural cell transplants (GEC, 2011). The Council adopted a three-tiered approach to research oversight, stating that neural cell transplants made by the transfer of human cells into mammals other than primates is ethically acceptable if the objective of the research is of overriding importance to medically benefit humanity, the generally applicable ethical requirements of animal welfare are satisfied, and the human cells are transferred after the embryonic stage. A second tier of research, including research involving the transplantation of human cells into nonhuman primate brains, should undergo rigorous review by a national-level committee. The Council recommended that a national-level committee already established for the use of animals in research be tasked with oversight of these types of studies, and that particularly rigorous review be applied to research that may result in changes in the capabilities of an animal that are relevant to its moral status. Studies involving transplantation of human stem cells into the brains of great apes fall into the third tier and should be prohibited. The Embryo Protection Act of 1990 had essentially already placed fusion of nonhuman animal embryos with human embryos into the third tier by prohibiting this research.[36]

The United Kingdom Home Office adopted guidance of this type in 2016 in response to a report from the UK Academy of Medical Sciences (Academy of Medical Sciences, 2011). The policy lists three categories of research: (1) experiments that do not present issues beyond those of the general use of animals in research and should be carried out under the normal regulatory structures that govern other types of animal research; (2) experiments that are permissible pending specialist review by the Animals in Science Committee, a national expert body; and (3) a narrow range of experiments that should not be licensed because of a lack of scientific justification or very strong ethical concerns. Experiments that fall into the second tier (which require national-level review) include "substantial modification of an animal's brain that may make the brain function potentially more 'human-like', particularly in large animals; experiments that may lead to the generation or propagation of functional human germ cells in animals; experiments that could be expected to significantly alter the appearance or behaviour of animals, affecting those characteristics that are perceived to contribute most to distinguishing our species from our close evolutionary relatives; and experiments involving the addition of human genes or cells to nonhuman primates (NHPs)." Experiments in the third tier (which should be prohibited) include "allowing the development of an embryo, formed by pre-implantation mixing of NHP and human embryonic or pluripotent stem cells, beyond 14 days of development or the first signs of primitive streak development (whichever occurs first); unless there is persuasive evidence that the fate of the implanted (human) cells will not lead to 'sensitive' phenotypic changes in the developing fetus; transplantation of sufficient

---

[36] German Embryo Protection Act (October 24, 1990). § 7(1) of the Act prohibits, among other things, combining embryos with different genetic information to form a cluster of cells, using at least one human embryo. See https://www.bundesgesundheitsministerium.de/fileadmin/Dateien/3_Downloads/Gesetze_und_Verordnungen/GuV/E/ESchG_EN_Fassung_Stand_10Dez2014_01.pdf.

human-derived neural cells into an NHP as to make it possible, in the judgement of the national expert body, that there could be substantial functional modification of the NHP brain, such as to engender 'human-like' behaviour. . . ; and breeding of animals that have, or may develop, human derived germ cells in their gonads, where this could lead to the production of human embryos or true hybrid embryos within an animal."[37] Canadian science-funding agencies issued a policy statement in 2018 that also follows this three-tiered approach. It states that grafting or transferring of hPSCs into a nonhuman animal after birth is permitted for certain applications,[38] but requires approval from an institutional research ethics board (similar to an IRB) and the Stem Cell Oversight Committee, a national-level committee under the auspices of the Canadian Institutes of Health Research. Prohibited research includes studies in which hESCs, embryonic germ cells, iPSCs, or other cells that are likely to be pluripotent are combined with or grafted or transferred to a nonhuman embryo or fetus (CIHR et al., 2018).

In Japan, prior to 2019, researchers were forbidden to grow nonhuman animal embryos containing human cells beyond 14 days or to transplant human-animal chimeric embryos into a surrogate uterus. In March 2019, however, the Japanese Ministry of Science announced guidance allowing Japanese researchers to use blastocyst complementation to inject human iPSCs into a nonhuman animal embryo for basic research, to produce better models with which to study human development and disease, and to create potential donor organs. Although this guidance does not explicitly follow the three-tiered approach, it requires that researchers apply for approval from an institutional ethics committee and a national-level Japanese special committee for research ethics to conduct this type of research (Zimmer, 2019). The guidance neither explicitly allows nor prohibits the use of nonhuman primates, although research on great apes is not allowed in Japan.

The Swiss Federal Act on Assisted Reproduction,[39] enacted in 1998, forbids the introduction of hESCs into nonhuman animal embryos, but does not specifically address the introduction of human iPSCs (presumably because this scientific development was not anticipated at the time of enactment), leading to some confusion about whether such an experiment would be allowed (SAMS, 2009; Shaw, 2014). The Swiss National Advisory Committee on Biomedical Ethics (NEK) issued a report in 2006 addressing broader research involving the transplantation of human cells into nonhuman animals (NeK, 2007). The report highlighted concerns about transplantation into the brain, in part because the possibility of altered perception or consciousness of the animal could not be excluded. The majority

---

[37] UK Home Office, Guidance on the use of Human Material in Animals, Advice Note 01/16, January 2016 (available at https://www.gov.uk/government/publications/guidance-on-the-use-of-human-material-in-animals).

[38] These experiments are permitted provided that (1) they are designed to reconstitute a specific tissue or organ to derive a preclinical model or to demonstrate that the cells are pluripotent, and (2) these nonhuman animals grafted with human stem cells will not be used for reproductive purposes.

[39] The Swiss Federal Reproductive Medicine Act of December 18, 1998, SR 810.11, AS 2000 3055.

of the members of the NEK opposed the creation or formation of partial human structures within animal hosts because of the concern that the human-animal chimera would develop a rudimentary form of the perception, sensibility, experience, or consciousness of humans. A minority of members supported limited authorization if one could control the development of the host organism.

Oversight of research involving neural cell transplants and human neural chimeras in China is unclear. In 2003, the Ministry of Science and Technology and the Ministry of Health enacted the Ethical Guidelines for Research on Human Embryonic Stem Cells, which includes some oversight at the national and institutional levels for these cells (Liao et al., 2007), but it is not clear whether this oversight includes neural cell transplant or human-animal chimera research. Certainly, research of this type is moving forward in China. A team of U.S., Spanish, and Chinese researchers produced the first human-monkey chimera at the Chinese Academy of Sciences' Kunming Institute of Zoology in July 2019 (Lin, 2020).[40] In this study, human cells were added to a monkey embryo and allowed to mature for about a week (Regalado, 2019).

FUTURE OVERSIGHT

Issues Regarding Consent

As discussed above, human biospecimens and data used in research are commonly "deidentified," at which point the donors are no longer considered human subjects, and with the exception of ensuring that initial donation conditions are honored, Common Rule oversight will not apply. However, DNA sequencing techniques combined with data from other sources have increasingly allowed for the reidentification of biospecimens that do not have such explicit identifiers, as has occurred multiple times in criminal investigations and prosecutions (Ram et al., 2018). If such techniques become widespread or common, this situation will raise both practical and ethical concerns. As NIH leadership has recently written, "With increasingly sophisticated genomic sequencing technology, interoperable databases, and artificial intelligence/machine learning approaches, the concept of being able to 'deidentify' biospecimens for future research use—the critical regulatory delineation between needing consent or not—is rapidly becoming obsolete" (Wolinetz and Collins, 2020). In an effort to address concerns about reidentification, new methods are being devised that obscure tell-tale sequence variants without unduly compromising data required for the success of research (Gürsoy et al., 2020). Other new methods allow analysis by researchers requesting access to data while protecting the privacy of individuals whose genomes are in the dataset (see, e.g., Mott et al., 2020). On the other hand, this is a fast-moving

---

[40] The U.S. researcher on the team, Juan Carlos Izpisua Belmonte, is a professor at the Salk Institute for Biological Studies in San Diego, CA.

field, and it remains uncertain whether new data protection methods will be able to keep up with novel methods for reidentification.[41]

Another consent issue concerns potential future research with biospecimens. Because it is impossible to identify all potential future uses of biospecimens to be deposited in a biobank at the time informed consent is obtained, some have suggested an approach that places greater emphasis on an ongoing good governance model for the biobank than on initial consent for future uses of the biospecimens. O'Doherty and colleagues (2011) outline four principles for biobank governance intended to both protect participant interests and promote effective translational health research: (1) recognition of research participants and publics as a collective body, (2) trustworthiness, (3) adaptive management to reflect dynamic technologies or changes in the nature or purpose of the biobank over time, and (4) fit between the nature of a particular biobank and the specific structural elements of governance adopted (O'Doherty et al., 2011, 367–374). These principles form the basis for an adaptive governance framework.

Boers and Bredenoord (2018) also propose addressing future uses of research biospecimens within a governance framework. Rather than creating an exhaustive list of potential future uses (such as the use of tissues to create neural organoids), participants consent to donating tissue to a biobank with an explicitly described governance model. They agree to a broad range of research uses, subject to privacy protections; a biobank governance structure that addresses consent procedures, management of data and samples, withdrawal of consent, property rights, communication with donors, and commercial interests; ongoing engagement with participants and the public; and fair sharing of research benefits. When possible, information on foreseeable research projects or procedures can be provided at the time of initial consent, particularly if certain procedures are foreseen that are known to be sensitive, such as whole-genome sequencing or human-animal chimera research (Sugarman and Bredenoord, 2019).

Another potential model for incorporating a governance framework into biobank practices is the nonprofit UK Biobank,[42] which has an Ethics and Governance Framework and an Ethics Advisory Committee that advises the UK Biobank Board on ethical issues that arise during the maintenance, development, and use of the biobank's resources, including identifying relevant ethical issues and providing guidance on policies with ethical dimensions. The consent form[43] informs the donor of the biobank's practices but does not describe specific research uses.

Many bioethicists and other observers have argued, however, that some research raises ethical issues that may warrant specific informed consent when

---

[41] Data protection methods encompass other methods in addition to encryption, including those that slightly perturb datasets to decrease the risk of reidentification while preserving utility for secondary analyses.

[42] See https://www.ukbiobank.ac.uk.

[43] See https://www.ukbiobank.ac.uk/wp- content/uploads/2011/06/Consent_form.pdf?phpMyAdmin= trmKQlYdjjnQIgJ%2CfAzikMhEnx6.

donated tissues will be used for these types of studies. The National Academies Guidelines for Human Embryonic Stem Cell Research state that specific informed consent should be required when human stem cells are used for transplantation into nonhuman animals.[44] The ISSCR guidelines also recommend that researchers inform participants when their tissues might be used in this way,[45] and the state of California has a similar requirement for research funded by the state.[46] An interdisciplinary group of brain researchers and ethicists stated in 2018:

> Currently, researchers using pluripotent stem cells or brain tissues generally disclose their plans to donors in broad terms. Given how much people associate their experiences and sense of self with their brains, more transparency and assurances could be warranted. Donors might wish to deny the use of their stem cells for the creation of, say, human–animal chimaeras" (Farahany et al., 2018).

With regard to procurement of human biological materials for neural organoid research, Hyun and colleagues (2020) write that donors should be informed that neural organoids will be generated. According to these authors, when researchers generate neural organoids using iPSC lines derived from deidentified tissue samples procured from tissue banks, "It cannot be assumed that tissue donors have given their consent for their participation specifically in brain organoid research" (Hyun et al., 2020).

The NIH Clinical Center's Department of Bioethics convened a workshop in 2015 for bioethics scholars on the topic of broad consent for research with biological samples (Grady et al., 2015). The workshop, which predated the final changes to the Common Rule, considered the ethical acceptability of broad consent for future research on stored biospecimens. Workshop participants concluded that broad consent is generally appropriate for use of biospecimens in repositories but may not be appropriate for exceptional circumstances. Examples of the latter included research proposing to create gametes from iPSCs or engaging certain donor groups, such as those with rare or highly stigmatized disorders or indigenous groups. Research on neural organoids or transplantation of human cells into nonhuman animals was not specifically discussed in this workshop.

Animal Welfare

If the acquisition of new capacities is suspected in animals used in research involving neural transplants or chimeras, additional training may be needed for

---

[44] NRC and IOM, 2010, §§ 3.6 and 7.1.
[45] ISSCR, 2016, Appendix 1.
[46] California Institute of Regenerative Medicine Regulations, Cal. Code Regs. Title 17 § 100100 (Informed Consent Requirements).

evaluators. Some of those responsible for oversight for research animals believe that plans could be developed for species-specific needs that would take into account previous experience with the domesticated species, the behavior of the wild population, the needs of similar species, and preference testing (i.e., tests to determine which conditions and environments the animals prefer). If warranted, an IACUC could authorize a pilot program or require veterinary evaluations. Ensuring the welfare of a laboratory animal includes ongoing monitoring after the research has been approved for behaviors (such as those related to activity, feeding, and socializing) and sometimes physiological parameters (such as blood pressure, heart rate, and cortisol levels) that are not typical of the individual or the species. Researchers work with the attending veterinarian to address any concerns—for example, by adjusting the animal's diet or caging or changing the experimental protocol. In addition, as discussed below, IACUCs could gain additional expertise on animal welfare from animal ethologists and animal behavior scientists if needed.

Addition of Ad Hoc Expertise

The existing institutional oversight committees for human neural organoid, transplant, and chimera research have specific regulatory charges, such as protection of human subjects for IRBs and animal welfare for IACUCs. If these local committees lacked sufficient expertise to review research studies on the topics discussed in this report, they could add members with relevant expertise—for example, in stem cell research, neurobiology, species-specific behaviors and needs, and animal ethics or religious studies. These members could join on an ad hoc basis. If needed, experts from other institutions could participate in meetings via videoconference.

Further Discussion of Oversight as the Research Develops

As is clear from the previous chapter, the research discussed in this report may invoke much broader ethical concerns that do not fall within the expertise or scope of these existing committees. As research involving human neural organoids, transplants, and chimeras advances, there may be additional opportunities at the national level for discussion of ethical issues and oversight. For example, the Novel and Exceptional Technology and Research Advisory Committee (NExTRAC) is a potential U.S. forum for future discussions on the ethical and regulatory issues associated with these research models. A successor to the Recombinant DNA Advisory Committee (RAC), NExTRAC was established in 2019 as a federal advisory committee to the director of NIH. It is tasked with making recommendations on the scientific, safety, ethical, and social issues associated with areas of emerging biotechnology research, but does not review individual protocols. As the new NExTRAC framework is being developed to evaluate emerging biotechnologies or applications,[47] one NExTRAC priority will be to advise NIH on effective communication and outreach on emerging biotechnologies. Research involving human neural organoids, transplants, and chimeras might be an appropriate topic for NExTRAC consideration if requested by the NIH director. As an advisory committee, however, NExTRAC can only offer recommendations to NIH leadership, who then must decide whether to accept and implement them.

NIH has also used workshops (such as those mentioned above) and expert committees with narrower purview to gain helpful insight into complex topics. For example, the Neuroethics Subgroup of the BRAIN Initiative has provided guidance relevant to ethical issues in neuroscience.[48] Such venues can provide timely and highly relevant perspectives. More broadly, the U.S. government has used multiple types of entities to provide insight on bioethical issues. Congress established two bioethics commissions: the National Commission for the Protection of Human Subjects of Biomedical and Behavioral Research (1974–1978) and the President's Commission for the Study of Ethical Problems in Medicine and Biomedical and Behavioral Research (1980–1983). In addition, each U.S. president from 1996 to 2016 appointed a bioethics council or commission to study scientific issues with ethical dimensions. The National Bioethics Advisory Commission (1996–2001),[49] the President's Bioethics Council (2001–2009), and the Presidential Commission for the Study of Bioethical Issues (2009–2017) released reports on such issues as stem cell research (PCB, 2004), human cloning (PCB, 2002), human research subjects (PCSBI, 2011), and topics in neuroscience (PCSBI, 2015). Although these activities can be valuable, they are sometimes seen as guided in part by political influence because their members are appointed by the President. As mentioned throughout the present report, reports commissioned from the National Academies have also been influential in these discussions as offering consensus, peer-reviewed expert perspectives. Whether these mechanisms, separately or in combination, are useful for dealing with ethical issues that might be raised by these kinds of research in the future is beyond the scope of this report.

---

[47] See https://osp.od.nih.gov/biotechnology/main-nextrac/#activities.
[48] See https://acd.od.nih.gov/working-groups/brain2.0-subgroup.html.
[49] See https://bioethicsarchive.georgetown.edu/nbac/pubs.html.

5

Public Engagement

Public engagement can be defined in various ways, adopt various formats, and have various goals (NASEM, 2017a).[1] Some activities are designed as one-way communication from researchers to the public, while others are designed as "conversations that support two-way learning" (Staley and Barron, 2019) or "dialogues of science, ethics and religion."[2] The formats include, among others, focus groups, testimony at hearings, community advisory groups, and consultations. Goals include educating the public, informing the public about research studies, disseminating research findings, seeking advice, providing input for policy making, increasing research participation, establishing dialogue, and increasing trust. Robust public engagement is important when sensitive new biotechnologies emerge and even more important when research on these technologies is publicly funded. Implementing public engagement presents challenges, including how to select individuals and groups to participate, how to help participants understand the scientific issues and existing regulations and oversight, and how to respond to controversy or public opposition.

PUBLIC ENGAGEMENT INTERNATIONALLY AND IN THE UNITED STATES

Other countries have national procedures and institutions in place to facilitate public engagement. The United Kingdom has Sciencewise,[3] a semi-independent

---

[1] See https://www.aaas.org/programs/dialogue-science-ethics-and-religion.
[2] Dietram Scheufele, University of Wisconsin–Madison, presentation to committee, October 29, 2020, virtual meeting. PNAS paper, in press.
[3] See Scheufele et al., 2021.

government agency intended to facilitate such public engagement, including through polling, deliberative dialog, and written consultations.[4] The United Kingdom has also used "citizen assemblies" to discuss complex issues such as climate change.[5] The UK Academy of Medical Sciences conducted a public consultation in the process of producing its 2011 report *Animals Containing Human Materials* (Academy of Medical Sciences, 2011); however, the process and the summary of its findings have been criticized (Baylis, 2009). Denmark has "a longstanding tradition of consensus conferences for which broad representation is sought, and whose results are taken seriously in the policy-making process" (NASEM, 2017a). This process is coordinated by a government agency, the Danish Board of Technology. The United States currently lacks effective mechanisms to facilitate or carry out public engagement at the national level. At the local level, a prominent genetics researcher has established a project designed to inform diverse communities about genomics through workshops in schools, faith communities, libraries, museums, youth groups, and community spaces (Marcus, 2018).

The void in public engagement in the United States has been noted, and several National Academies' reports and activities have called for greater public engagement with emerging innovative areas of biotechnology and biomedical research. For example, the 2017 National Academies report on human genome editing (NASEM, 2017a) calls for public engagement, participation, and input in policy development, particularly before approval of research that includes genome edits that are heritable or go beyond prevention or treatment of disease. Statements from the organizing committees for two International Summits on Human Genome Editing organized by the National Academies also call for such engagement (NASEM, 2015, 2019b). The 2016 report *Gene Drives on the Horizon* includes extensive guidance and recommendations on stakeholder engagement (NASEM, 2016a). Other reports call for public engagement on other biotechnologies, including those focused on mitochondrial replacement techniques (NASEM, 2016c), genetically engineered crops (NASEM, 2016b), and novel biotechnology products (NASEM, 2017b, 2019a) to help inform future directions. However, these recommendations for public engagement have not been broadly implemented. The committee notes that in the United States, regardless of public attitudes and values, there are other considerations in play in setting policy, including constitutional limitations on what government can do to abridge freedoms.

Public engagement strategies must be based on the realization that many people base their reactions to biotechnological innovations, including human neural organoid, transplant, and chimera research, on core beliefs and values that commonly are grounded in their religious beliefs. In the United States, there are a wide range of religious perspectives and multiple views within any faith tradi-

---

[4] Robin Lovell-Badge, Francis Crick Institute, presentation to committee, November 13, 2020, virtual meeting.

[5] See https://www.climateassembly.uk.

tion. At the same time, many people base their core beliefs on secular values, which also are diverse. The committee found that engaging in discussions with experts in medicine, biology, philosophy, law, theology, religious studies, and other disciplines was very useful. Based on its experience, the committee believes that such discussions can be mutually enlightening and might be even more so if they were sustained over multiple meetings or over an extended period of time.

Because of the plurality of religious and secular views in the United States concerning biotechnological innovations, respectful dialogues between religious and secular perspectives and among different viewpoints could help build mutual understanding. Even if individuals from different disciplines, communities, and faith traditions do not reach agreement on specific policies, it is useful for each group to feel that they have been listened to and understood by others. For example, speakers from disciplines other than science who addressed the committee were interested in learning about the research discussed in the report. Such discussions might also build an appreciation of why other people hold different views, find common ground, and forge connections and trust.

There are many unresolved questions about how respectful dialogues and discussions might be carried out: What should be the goals? Who should convene them? What format should be used? Is it useful to have people meet over an extended period of time or in several sessions? Under what circumstances would it be desirable to hold them locally, regionally, or nationally? The answers to these questions will likely vary on the basis of topic and the purpose of the discussions. It will be useful to learn from various types of public engagement that have been carried out on various topics—What were the strengths, weaknesses, and lessons learned?

POTENTIAL CONTRIBUTION OF SOCIAL SCIENCE RESEARCH

In addition to public engagement, social science research, ultimately building to a representative sample of the U.S. population, could identify public attitudes regarding human neural organoids, transplants, and chimeras and contribute to oversight policy. Unfortunately, the committee was unable to find documentation of research specific to these topics. There have been empirical studies of public attitudes regarding nonneural chimeras, such as pigs with organs compatible with humans that could be transplanted to humans, although these studies were not done with a representative sample of the U.S. population.

A population-based U.S. survey on genetic engineering, a topic that also raises public concerns, found that "most Americans accept genetic engineering of animals that benefits human health, but many oppose other uses" (Funk and Hefferon, 2018). When asked about producing "animals to grow organs/tissues for humans needing a transplant," 41 percent said that this would be "taking technology too far," and 57 percent said it would be an "appropriate use of technology." This study also found that 52 percent of Americans opposed the use of animals in research; more people were opposed to chimeric than to other animals (69 percent vs. 47 percent). It is possible that there would be still more opposition to neural chimeras generated for purposes other than organ or tissue donation, which was the topic of this survey. Surveys addressing this issue could help inform public policy.

It is also important to know *why* groups in the public support or oppose particular types of research, information that can be used to determine whether technology can proceed in ways that support the values of the public. In the survey of genetic engineering, a qualitative follow-up question explored objections to chimeric animals for organ transplantation. A range of objections was elicited: 21 percent of objections were coded as focused on animal suffering, 11 percent on "messing with God's plan," 6 percent on "messing with nature," 16 percent on human health, and 9 percent on unintended consequences in general, with smaller percentages focused on other concerns. Well-designed research on the public's attitudes toward human neural organoids, transplants, and chimeras, as well as on why they hold those attitudes and which groups have specific reasons, would help inform policies regarding this research. As discussed in Chapter 3, ethical implications are sometimes associated with a "yuck" factor, which can be difficult for individuals to delineate logically. Even so, such feelings can erode trust in the scientific process if they are not identified and addressed in engagement and discussion.

NOMENCLATURE

When conducting any type of public engagement, it is important to choose nomenclature carefully. Kathleen Hall Jamieson, a professor of communication, discussed with the committee the implications of terms used to describe innovative biotechnology. Jamieson said that all can agree on the importance of scientific accuracy. She also cautioned that some terms may induce listeners to bring to bear concerns and associations from other, unrelated debates. She advised that words used to describe new research should not lead listeners to draw false inferences or attempt to persuade them that the innovative science is desirable. Instead, Jamieson suggested that a good term should induce the listener to want to learn more about the science.[6]

In this report, therefore, the committee uses the terms "neural organoid," "neural transplant," and "neural chimera" not only because they are scientifically accurate and widely used to denote these research models but also because they do not represent an attempt to lead the reader to a conclusion and are not connected to unrelated ethical debates. Likewise, the committee eschewed such terms as "mini-brain" because they are scientifically inaccurate and may also

---

[6] Kathleen Hall Jamieson, University of Pennsylvania's Annenberg School for Communication, presentation to the committee, July 15, 2020, virtual meeting.

lead members of the public to perceive that ethical boundaries have been crossed when in reality they have not. Such terms as "humanized" were also avoided because in this case, the term implies that a nonhuman animal could or has become human, thus invoking a stance in the ethical debate about what it means to be human. The term "chimera" is used because it is scientifically accurate, and the committee believes that its connection with the monsters of ancient myths is too remote to warrant avoiding its use. Research scientists and their institutional representatives can be cautioned to avoid terminology that may court attention but does their work a disservice by stimulating concerns that go far beyond the current state of the science.

6

Findings of the Committee

The committee's findings fall into six areas:

1. Value of this research
2. State of the science
3. Issues of ethical concern
4. Assessment of consciousness and pain in human neural organoids, transplants, and chimeras
5. Oversight and regulation
6. Public engagement and communication

VALUE OF THIS RESEARCH

Finding I.1: Brain diseases—neurological and psychiatric disorders—are the leading cause of morbidity worldwide, resulting in mortality and untold suffering, as well as enormous financial burdens in health care costs and lost wages. There are few if any highly effective treatments for many of these disorders, which include traumatic injury; neurodegenerative diseases, such as Alzheimer's disease, Parkinson's disease, and amyotrophic lateral sclerosis; psychiatric diseases, such as schizophrenia and bipolar disorder; developmental disorders, such as autism spectrum disorder; and brain cancers. The lack of progress in developing therapeutics for these disorders in large part reflects a lack of knowledge regarding the underlying disease processes in the developing or adult brain and how brain aging contributes to disease onset and progression. The development of new therapies will require a foundation of greater basic knowledge about human brain development, maturation, and function and greater translational knowledge about the mechanisms of brain diseases. However, research on the human brain itself is limited by a combination of legal, practical, and ethical restrictions, as well as technical hurdles. Small animal models provide a valuable alternative, but they are insufficient for studying complex human brain disorders.

Finding I.2: Recent advances in human stem cell research now enable ready access to human neurons and glial cells, facilitating the development of more sophisticated models with which to study brain diseases and disorders in greater depth. Human neural organoids, transplants, and chimeras are powerful models that use stem cells to circumvent many of the limitations noted above, providing novel ways to understand normal and abnormal human brain development, analyze disease mechanisms, and assess therapeutic approaches. Thus, they have the potential to be invaluable additions to human studies and animal models. The promise of these novel human brain cell models is that they will contribute to understanding of the mechanisms of brain development and function, and pave the way for the development of transformative therapies that can relieve the significant burden of neurological and psychiatric diseases. However, this promise must be carefully weighed against the ethical concerns such models may raise.

State of the Science

Finding II.1: Human neural organoids are cellular aggregates derived from human stem cells, in which multiple, diverse types of neuronal and glial cells differentiate and form three-dimensional organized assemblies. They have been used to model several aspects of human brain development and structure. Organoids generated from patient-derived stem cells sometimes exhibit disease phenotypes that can be used to elucidate pathogenic mechanisms and test potential interventions. However, organoids are limited in size and complexity and lack important cell types, brain regions, and anatomically organized neural circuits thought to be required for complex human brain function, including consciousness. Researchers are actively pursuing new techniques for overcoming these limitations of organoids, and this work will likely lead to organoids of increased size and greater complexity. Maturation is also likely to be improved, but the likelihood of generating a structure with the intricate organization, wealth of diverse cell types, and complex interconnectedness that would resemble in any significant way the mature functioning human brain is remote for the foreseeable future.

Finding II.2: Transplantation of human neural cells into the brains of nonhuman animals shows promise for improving models of neurological and psychiatric disease. Human glial precursors can be introduced into the brain of animal models, where they differentiate, integrate, and function. However, limitations exist that determine the level of maturation and integration of the transplanted cells within the host brain. These limitations are due to species-specific differences in developmental times whereby, for example, human brain cells mature much more slowly than their mouse counterparts, even upon transplantation in the mouse brain. The result is a developmental mismatch that is likely to affect the contribution of human neural cells to the working circuits of the host.

In chimeric animals (as defined above), donor and host cells develop together from the earliest stages of embryogenesis. In one such method, blastocyst complementation, host cells that would normally contribute to particular brain regions are eliminated at an early stage, allowing extensive replacement of those regions by donor cells. To date, neural chimeras generated by these methods use donor and host cells from the same or closely related species. It is not currently possible to generate neural chimeras of human cells in embryos of any nonhuman species that survive postnatally or even to late fetal stages. Generation of such chimeras may eventually be more feasible in nonhuman primates than in rodents.

Issues of Ethical Concern

Finding III.1: Because of the human suffering and mortality caused by brain disorders, limitations of current animal disease models, and the uniquely human quality of some brain diseases, there are strong moral arguments in favor of research using organoids, transplants, and chimeras derived from human cells as long as such research is balanced with other ethical considerations, such as ensuring animal welfare, appropriate use of human biological materials, and safety.

Finding III.2: Some studies in which human neural cells have been integrated into the brains of nonhuman animals raise moral, ethical, and religious concerns regarding the mixing of humans and other animals, the special status of humans, animals acquiring attributes that could be viewed as distinctively human, or humans taking on roles that should be reserved for a deity. Similar objections may also be raised from a secular viewpoint—for example, that conducting such research shows hubris or that the resulting entity offends the dignity of human beings.

A key concern is that a fundamental distinction between humans and other animals could be blurred. The increasing ability to generate human-animal chimeras with greater integration of human neural cells heightens this concern. There may also be concerns that some human cells outside the body should not be treated as mere clumps of matter. Some types of cells, such as human blastocysts and embryonic stem cells that are considered potential or actual human beings, are accorded greater or special respect, depending on one's religious and philosophical views.

Finding III.3: Under Subpart A of the Federal Policy for the Protection of Human Subjects, often called the Common Rule, existing biological materials that have been collected with appropriate consent and deidentified may be used in future research projects. However, provisions of the Common Rule are seen by some as a minimal standard for meeting ethical requirements in this area. For biological materials collected in the past, specific consent for human neural organoid, transplant, and chimera research was generally not obtained. There is active discussion regarding the advantages and disadvantages of obtaining specific consent going forward for the collection of fresh tissue for such research.

As a practical matter, recontacting donors to obtain specific consent is sometimes impossible. Moreover, many induced pluripotent stem cell (iPSC) lines obtained from donor tissue have been extensively characterized or were derived from patients with very rare diseases, and deriving new lines would be extremely difficult in these cases. On the other hand, most donors were not aware that their tissues would be used for neural organoid, cell transplant, or chimera research, and some might have objected if directly asked for their consent for such uses. Past ethics violations during research with African American and Native American participants make this a sensitive topic for these populations.

Finding III.4: Nonhuman animals have interests and some believe they have rights. Humans should therefore respect their well-being and their intrinsic nature and telos. However, there is wide agreement that it is permissible to use animals for basic and translational research directed toward the goal of relieving human suffering as long as the research is justified in terms of prospective benefit to human health, harm to animals is minimized, and the needs of the animals are met. Well-established regulations and practices emphasize the requirements to minimize the number of animals used; replace them with other experimental models when possible and consistent with the approved scientific aims of the research; alleviate or minimize their pain and distress; and provide them appropriate living conditions, including nutritious food, safe shelter, housing, companionship, and opportunities for stimulation.

As transplantation and chimeric models of human brain diseases become better able to model key disease features, research animals are likely to show behaviors that resemble human symptoms and that would be viewed as distressing were they to occur in humans. Close observation of the animals can identify such behaviors, which may need to be avoided or mitigated to maintain animal welfare. Another concern is that host animals might acquire altered behaviors wholly atypical of their species, such as new forms of problem solving or substantially altered, complex social interactions. If so, objections to using such animals for research might increase. The committee found scant evidence that this is a realistic possibility in the foreseeable future, but surveillance of this rapidly developing research is essential.

Finding III.5: The complexity of neural organoids is currently limited. It is extremely unlikely that in the foreseeable future they would possess capacities that, given current understanding, would be recognized as awareness, consciousness, emotion, or the experience of pain. Thus, it appears at present that neural organoids have no more moral standing than other in vitro human neural tissues or cultures. As scientists develop significantly more complex organoids, however, the need to make this distinction will need to be revisited regularly. Moreover, organoids can be transplanted into the brain, blurring the distinction between organoids and transplants.

Assessment of Consciousness and Pain in Human Neural Organoids, Transplants, and Chimeras

Finding IV.1: Decisions about how research on neural cell transplantation and chimeras should be conducted or overseen depend in large part on the possibility that the animal host will have altered capacities as a consequence of its brain cells being augmented or replaced by human cells. The possibilities of pain sensation, and altered consciousness are often raised as issues of particular concern, but both pain and consciousness are difficult to define or measure. While measurements of neuronal activity and circuit physiology are possible in organoids, these measurements are not considered sufficient to determine whether organoids may be conscious or feel pain. In contrast, when human cells are incorporated in a host brain, via either chimera formation or cell transplantation, it will be possible to devise and deploy methods for detecting differences in the behavior of that host compared with that of a host in which human cells have not been integrated. Some metrics and indicators already exist, particularly for pain. Likewise, there are quantitative methods for assessing behavior with high temporal and spatial resolution. Research veterinarians, ethologists, and animal behavior researchers are well suited to providing guidance on how to identify and interpret behaviors that are not typical of the species or the individual.

Finding IV.2: Most current methods for assessing consciousness (sometimes called awareness or sentience) and pain cannot be applied to organoids because understanding of these capacities depends largely on observing behaviors in whole animals. With the current state of knowledge, it would be difficult to use these measurements as evidence for the existence of pain or consciousness in organoids.

Oversight and Regulation

Finding V.1: Many ethical concerns raised by current and near-future research can be addressed by current oversight mechanisms, which are often created for specific ethical purposes. Nonetheless, some concerns will need be reassessed as the science develops.

Finding V.2: Neural organoids will not raise issues that require additional oversight until and unless they become significantly more complex.

Finding V.3: Transplantation of human neural cells or human neural organoids into nonhuman animals falls under a well-developed oversight system for animal research. In the United States, this system is built on the Animal Welfare Act and the Public Health Service Policy on Humane Care and Use of Laboratory Animals (PHS Policy). It includes review and approval of research protocols by institutional animal care and use committees (IACUCs), as well as on-the-ground monitoring by research veterinarians and animal caregivers. As currently constituted, however, some IACUCs may not contain sufficient independent expertise in neural cell transplant or chimera research or interpretation of animal behavior after transplantation of human neural cells.

Finding V.4: The animal welfare concerns raised by the generation of neural chimeras through blastocyst complementation in rodents also fall under significant and capable oversight by IACUCs and research veterinarians. Again, however, additional expertise on topics such as behavioral capabilities may be required.

Finding V.5: Some future research, including that involving more complex human neural organoids, transplants, and chimeras and the generation of transplants and chimeras in nonhuman primates, will benefit from additional discussion of ethical and social issues that extend beyond reviews of individual research projects currently carried out by IACUCs. Examples include injection of human stem cells into nonhuman animal blastocysts and indications that suggest enhanced capacities in transplant recipients or chimeras. Possibilities for additional oversight or safeguards include pilot studies followed by re-evaluation, implementation of novel measures to monitor capacities of research animals, and designation of research that should not be conducted at this time. There are advantages to carrying out such discussions at the national level, where a wide range of viewpoints and disciplinary backgrounds could be convened.

Finding V.6: Interdisciplinary research organizations, such as the International Society for Stem Cell Research (ISSCR), periodically analyze the updated state of the science, but no national or governmental bodies in the United States have this task as part of their mandate. Moreover, there is currently no national body in the United States whose charge is to review emerging science in key areas or to assess their ethical and regulatory implications.

Finding V.7: In several fields of innovative and rapidly developing biomedical research that raise social and ethical concerns, such as human embryonic stem cell research and human genome editing, a three-tiered system of oversight has been recommended and, in some cases, adopted:

- research that can be carried out under current oversight procedures,
- research that requires heightened oversight, and
- research that should not be carried out at this time.

This system allows ethically uncontroversial research projects to be carried out without imposing an administrative burden while providing additional scrutiny of research projects for which attention to emergent issues or additional expertise in the review body is helpful.

Prohibition of some types of research can reflect widely accepted limits on research that have been articulated by public and scientific groups. A prohibition on conducting such research at present also allows for later reconsideration once the science has matured enough to understand its consequences, along with an updated assessment of ethical considerations.

Public Engagement and Communication

Finding VI.1: Calls have been increasing for greater public engagement in assessing the value of emerging areas of biomedical research. Such engagement has several benefits, including helping the public understand the research, identifying public concerns, facilitating informed public discussion, and influencing science policy. However, the United States currently lacks robust mechanisms for facilitating this public engagement. Analysis of lessons learned from efforts on related topics could support the design of effective strategies for engaging the public in discussion of human neural organoids, transplants, and chimeras.

Finding VI.2: Well-designed social science research could also help scientists, regulators, and policy makers better understand the views of the public. Social science research on public attitudes toward and perspectives on human neural organoid and chimera research is currently lacking in the United States.

Finding VI.3: During its meetings and deliberations, the committee appreciated hearing the perspectives of religious scholars of several faith traditions and engaging in discussions with experts in medicine, biology, philosophy, law, theology, religious studies, and other disciplines. These discussions were mutually enlightening and should be continued. Because of the plurality of religious and secular views in the United States, ongoing dialogues between religious and secular perspectives and among different viewpoints are important. There are currently few if any established forums for fostering this exchange.

Finding VI.4: In some cases, terms used to describe human neural organoids, transplants, and chimeras have been inaccurate, inadequately descriptive, or misleading. These terms can evoke, intentionally or unintentionally, emotional responses that do not reflect the science being described, and they can be used to pull the public toward acceptance or rejection of a technology. As one of many examples, neural organoids are often referred to in the press as "mini-brains," but in reality, they model only some limited aspects of brain tissue. Closer attention to issues of nomenclature by scientists and their institutional representatives in their interactions with the press and public would facilitate a more informed public debate about brain research.

References

Aach, J., J. Lunshof, E. Iyer, and G. M. Church. 2017, March 21. Addressing the ethical issues raised by synthetic human entities with embryo-like features. *eLife*. doi: 10.7554/eLife.20674.

AAMC (Association of American Medical Colleges). 2020, February 21. NIH convenes workshop on research rigor and reproducibility with nonhuman primates. https://www.aamc.org/advocacy-policy/washington-highlights/nih-convenes-workshop-research-rigor-and-reproducibility-nonhuman-primates.

Academy of Medical Sciences. 2011. *Animals Containing Human Material*. https://acmedsci.ac.uk/policy/policy-projects/animals-containing-human-material.

Adolphs, R., and D. J. Anderson. 2018. *The neuroscience of emotion: A new synthesis*. Princeton, NJ: Princeton University Press. doi: 10.23943/9781400889914.

Albanese, A., J. M. Swaney, D. H. Yun, N. B. Evans, J. M. Antonucci, S. Velasco, C. H. Sohn, P. Arlotta, L. Gehrke, and K. Chung. 2020. Multiscale 3D phenotyping of human cerebral organoids. *Scientific Reports* 10(1):21487. doi: 10.1038/S41598-020-78130-7.

Alves, P. N., C. Foulon, V. Karolis, D. Bzdok, D. S. Margulies, E. Volle, and M. T. de Schotten. 2019. An improved neuroanatomical model of the default-mode network reconciles previous neuroimaging and neuropathological findings. *Communications Biology* 2(370). doi: 10.1038/s42003-019-0611-3.

Andersen, J., O. Revah, Y. Miura, N. Thom, N. D. Amin, K. W. Kelley, M. Singh, X. Chen, M. V. Thete, E. M. Walczak, H. Vogel, H. C. Fan, and S. P. Paşca. 2020. Generation of functional human 3D cortico-motor assembloids. *Cell* 7(13):1913-1929.e26. doi: 10.1016/j.cell.2020.11.017.

Anderson, D. J., and R. Adolphs. 2014. A framework for studying emotions across species. *Cell* 157(1):187-200.

Anderson, J. R., and G. G. Gallup Jr. 2015. Mirror self-recognition: A review and critique of attempts to promote and engineer self-recognition in primates. *Primates* 56:317-326.

ASP (American Society of Primatologists). 2020. *Principles for ethical treatment of non-human primates*. Last revised July 6, 2020. https://www.asp.org/society/resolutions/EthicalTreatmentOfNonHumanPrimates.cfm.

AVMA (American Veterinary Medical Association). 2020. *Guidelines for the Euthanasia of Animals: 2020 edition*. Schaumberg, IL: American Veterinary Medical Association.

Baylis, F. 2009. The HFEA public consultation process on hybrids and chimeras: Informed, effective and meaningful. *Kennedy Institute of Ethics Journal* 19(1):41-62.

Baylis, F., and J. S. Robert. 2007. Part-human chimeras: Worrying the facts, probing the ethics. *American Journal of Bioethics* 7(5):41-45. doi: 10.1080/15265160701290397.

Beauchamp, T. L., and D. DeGrazia. 2020. *Principles of animal research ethics*. New York: Oxford University Press.

Bhaduri, A., M. G. Andrews, W. M. Leon, D. Jung, D. Shin, D. Allen, D. Jung, G. Schmunk, M. Haeussler, J. Salma, A. A. Pollen, T. J. Nowakowski, and A. R. Kriegstein. 2020. Cell stress in cortical organoids impairs molecular subtype specification. *Nature* 578(7793):142-148. doi: 10.1038/s41586-020-1962-0.

Birey, F., J. Andersen, C. Makinson, S. Islam, W. Wei, N. Huber, H. C. Fan, K. Cordes Metzler, G. Panagiotakos, N. Thom, N. O'Rourke, L. Steinmetz, J. Bernstein, J. Hallmayer, J. Huguenard, and S. Paşca. 2017. Assembly of functionally integrated human forebrain spheroids. *Nature* 545: 54-59. doi: 10.1038/nature22330.

Björklund, A., and O. Lindvall. 2000. Cell replacement therapies for central nervous system disorders. *Nature Neuroscience* 3(6):537-544. doi: 10.1038/75705.

Boers, S. N., and A. L. Bredenoord. 2018. Consent for governance in the ethical use of organoids. *Nature Cell Biology* 20: 642-645. doi10.1038/s41556-018-0112-5.

Bolliger, G. 2016. Legal protection of animal dignity in Switzerland: Status quo and future perspectives. *Animal Law* 22: 311-395.

Bräuer, J., D. Hanus, S. Pika, R. Gray, and N. Uomini. 2020. Old and new approaches to animal cognition: There is not "one cognition." *Journal of Intelligence* 8(3):28. doi: 10.3390/jintelligence8030028.

Braz, J. M., A. Etlin, D. Juarez-Salinas, I. J. Llewellyn-Smith, and A. I. Basbaum. 2017. Rebuilding CNS inhibitory circuits to control chronic neuropathic pain and itch. *Progress in Brain Research* 231:87-105.

Bringmann, A., S. Syrbe, K. Görner, J. Kacza, M. Francke, P. Wiedemann, and A. Reichenbach. 2018. The primate fovea: Structure, function and development. *Progress in Retinal and Eye Research* 66:49-84. doi: 10.1016/j.preteyeres.2018.03.006. PMID: 29609042.

Cao, Y., J. P. Vacanti, K. T. Paige, J. Upton, and C. A. Vacanti. 1997. Transplantation of chondrocytes utilizing a polymer-cell construct to produce tissue-engineered cartilage in the shape of a human ear. *Plastic and Reconstructive Surgery* 100(2):297-302. doi: 10.1097/00006534-199708000-00001.

Carbone, L. 2019. Ethical and IACUC considerations regarding analgesia and pain management in laboratory rodents. *Comparative Medicine* 69(6):443-450. doi: 10.30802/AALAS-CM- 18-000149.

CARTA (Center for Academic Research and Training in Anthropology). n.d. Matrix of comparative anthropogeny. https://carta.anthropogeny.org/moca.

Casali, A.G., O. Gosseries, M. Rosanova, M. Boly, S. Sarasso, K. R. Casali, S. Casarotto, M.-A. Bruno, S. Laureys, G. Tononi, and M. Massimini. 2013. A theoretically based index of consciousness independent of sensory processing and behavior. *Science Translational Medicine* 15(198):105. doi: 10.1126/scitranslmed.3006294.

CCWG (Council of Councils Working Group on the Use of Chimpanzees in NIH-Supported Research). 2013. Report. https://dpcpsi.nih.gov/council/pdf/FNL_Report_WG_Chimpanzees.pdf

Chang, A., Z. Liang, H.-Q. Dai, A. Chapdelaine-Williams, N. Andrews, R. Bronson, B. Schwer, and F. Alt. 2018. Neural blastocyst complementation enables mouse forebrain organogenesis. *Nature* 563:126-130. doi: 10.1038/s41586-018-0586-0.

Charo, R. A. 2006. Body of research—Ownership and use of human tissue. *New England Journal of Medicine* 355:1517-1519. doi: 10.1056/NEJMp068192.

CIHR (Canadian Institutes of Health Research), Natural Sciences and Engineering Research Council of Canada, and Social Sciences and Humanities Research Council. 2018. *Tri-council policy statement: Ethical conduct for research involving humans*. https://ethics.gc.ca/eng/policy-politique_tcps2-eptc2_2018.html.

REFERENCES

CIMS (Council for International Organization of Medical Sciences) and ICLAS (International Council for Laboratory Animal Science). 2012. *International guiding principles for biomedical research involving animals.* https://olaw.nih.gov/sites/default/files/Guiding_Principles_2012.pdf.
Clevers, H. 2016. Modeling development and disease with organoids. *Cell* 165(7):1586-1597.
Coghlan, A. 2014, December 1. The smart mouse with the half-human brain. *NewScientist.* https://www.newscientist.com/article/dn26639-the-smart-mouse-with-the-half-human-brain.
Cole-Turner, R. 1993. *The new Genesis: Theology and the genetic revolution*, 1st edition. Louisville, KY: Westminster John Knox Press.
Collins, F. 2015, November 17. NIH will no longer support biomedical research on chimpanzees. https://www.nih.gov/about-nih/who-we-are/nih-director/statements/nih-will-no-longer-support-biomedical-research-chimpanzees.
Comosy, C., and S. Kopp. 2014. The use of non-human animals in biomedical research: Can moral theology fill the gap? *Journal of Moral Theology* 3(2):54-71.
Cowan, C. S., M. Renner, M. De Gennaro, B. Gross-Scherf, D. Goldblum, Y. Hou, M. Munz, T. M. Rodrigues, J. Krol, T. Szikra, R. Cuttat, A. Waldt, P. Papasaikas, R. Diggelmann, C. P. Patino-Alvarez, P. Galliker, S. E. Spirig, D. Pavlinic, N. Gerber-Hollbach, S. Schuierer, A. Srdanovic, M. Balogh, R. Panero, A. Kusnyerik, A. Szabo, M. B. Stadler, S. Orgül, S. Picelli, P. W. Hasler, A. Hierlemann, H. P. N. Scholl, G. Roma, F. Nigsch, and B. Roska. 2020. Cell types of the human retina and its organoids at single-cell resolution. *Cell* 182(6):1623-1640.
Crawley, W. 2006, November 26. Peter Singer defends animal experimentation. BBC. https://www.bbc.co.uk/blogs/ni/2006/11/peter_singer_defends_animal_ex.html.
Cunningham, M., J.-H. Cho, A. Leung, G. Savvidis, S. Ahn, M. Moon, P. Lee, J. Han, N. Azimi, K.-S. Kim, V. Bolshakov, and S. Chung. 2014. hPSC-derived maturing GABAergic interneurons ameliorate seizures and abnormal behavior in epileptic mice. *Cell Stem Cell* 15:559-573.
Curtis, V. 2011. Why disgust matters. *Philosophical Transactions of the Royal Society B: Biological Sciences* 366(1583). doi: 10.1098/rstb.2011.0165.
D'Andola, M., B. Rebollo, A. G. Casali, J. F. Weinert, A. Pigorini, R. Villa, M. Massimini, and M. V. Sanchez-Vives. 2018. Bistability, causality, and complexity in cortical networks: An in vitro perturbational study. *Cerebral Cortex* 28(7):2233-2242. doi: 10.1093/cercor/bhx122.
De Cruz, H. and J. De Smedt. 2016. A natural history of natural theology. *Faith and Philosophy: Journal of the Society of Christian Philosophers* 33(3). DOI: 10.5840/faithphil201633367.
de Waal, F. B. M. 2019. Fish, mirrors, and a gradualist perspective on self-awareness. *PLOS Biology* 17(2):e3000112. doi: 10.1371/journal.pbio.3000112.
de Waal, F. B. M., and S. D. Preston. 2017. Mammalian empathy: Behavioural manifestations and neural basis. *Nature Reviews Neuroscience* 18(8):498-509. doi: 10.1038/nrn.2017.72.
DeGrazia, D. 2009. Self-awareness in animals. In *The Philosophy of Animal Minds*, edited by Robert W. Lurz. Cambridge: Cambridge University Press. Pp. 201-217.
Dehaene, S. 2014. *Consciousness and the brain: Deciphering how the brain codes our thoughts.* New York: Viking Press.
Del Dosso, A., J. P. Urenda, T. Nguyen, and G. Quadrato. 2020. Upgrading the physiological relevance of human brain organoids. *Neuron* 107(6):1014-1028.
Devlin, H. 2019, March 18. Scientists grow 'mini-brain on the move' that can contract muscle. *Guardian.* https://www.theguardian.com/science/2019/mar/18/scientists-grow-mini-brain-on-the-move-that-can-contract-muscle.
Devolder K., L. J. Yip, and T. Douglas. 2020, April 24. The ethics of creating and using human-animal chimeras. *Institute for Laboratory Animal Research Journal.* doi: 10.1093/ilar/ilaa002.
Disease and Injury Incidence and Prevalence Collaborators. 2018. Global, regional, and national incidence, prevalence, and years lived with disability for 354 diseases and injuries for 195 countries and territories, 1990-2017: A systematic analysis for the Global Burden of Disease Study 2017. *Lancet* 392:1789-1858.
Doerig, A., A. Schurger, and M. H. Herzog. 2020. Hard criteria for empirical theories of consciousness. *Cognitive Neuroscience* 12(2):41-62. doi: 1080/17588928.2020.1772214.

Driehuis, E., A. van Hoeck, K. Moore, S. Kolders, H. E. Francies, M. C. Gulersonmez, E. C. A. Stigter, B. Burgering, V. Geurts, A. Gracanin, G. Bounova, F. H. Morsink, R. Vries, S. Boj, J. van Es, G. J. A. Offerhaus, O. Kranenburg, M. J. Garnett, L. Wessels, E. Cuppen, L. A. A. Brosens, and H. Clevers. 2019. Pancreatic cancer organoids recapitulate disease and allow personalized drug screening. *Proceedings of the National Academy of Sciences* 116(52):26580-26590.

Edelman, D. B., B. J. Baars, and A.K. Seth. 2005. Identifying hallmarks of consciousness in non-mammalian species. *Consciousness and Cognition* 14(1):169-187. doi: 10.1016/j.concog.2004.09.001. PMID: 15766896.

Eiraku, M., K. Watanabe, M. Matsuo-Takasaki, M. Kawada, S. Yonemura, M. Matsumura, T. Wataya, A. Nishiyama, K. Muguruma, and Y. Sasai. 2008. Self-organized formation of polarized cortical tissues from ESCs and its active manipulation by extrinsic signals. *Cell Stem Cell* 3(5):519-532.

Eiraku, M., N. Takata, H. Ishibashi, M. Kawada, E. Sakakura, S. Okuda, K. Sekiguchi, T. Adachi, and Y. Sasai. 2011. Self-organizing optic-cup morphogenesis in three-dimensional culture. *Nature* 472(7341):51-56.

Esk, C., D. Lindenhofer, S. Haendeler, R. A. Wester, F. Pflug, B. Schroeder, J. A. Bagley, U. Elling, J. Zuber, A. von Haeseler, and J. A. Knoblich. 2020. A human tissue screen identifies a regulator of ER secretion as a brain size determinant. *Science* 370(6519):935-941. doi: 10.1126/science.abb5390.

Evans, J. H. 2016. *What is a human? What the answers mean for human rights.* New York: Oxford University Press.

Farahany, N. A., H. T. Greely, S. Hyman, C. Koch, C. Grady, S. P. Paşca, N. Sestan, P. Arlotta, J. L. Bernat, J. Ting, J. E. Lunshof, E. P. R. Iyer, I. Hyun, B. H. Capestany, G. M. Church, H. Huang, and H. Song. 2018. The ethics of experimenting with human brain tissue. *Nature* 556:429-432. doi: 10.1038/d41586-018-04813-x.

Feng, G., F. E. Jensen, H. T. Greely, H. Okano, S. Treue, A. C. Roberts, J. G. Fox, S. Caddick, M.-M. Poo, W. T. Newsome, and J. H. Morrison. 2020. Opportunities and limitations of genetically modified nonhuman primate models for neuroscience research. *Proceedings of the National Academy of Sciences* 117(39):24022-24031. doi: 10.1073/pnas.2006515117.

Fernandez, E. 2019, October 12. Minibrains grown in the laboratory produce brainwaves. now what? *Forbes*. https://www.forbes.com/sites/fernandezelizabeth/2019/10/12/minibrains-grown-in-the-laboratory-produce-brainwaves--now-what/?sh=4aab662f9ac7.

Filippi, M. 2015. *Oxford textbook of neuroimaging*, illustrated edition. Oxford Textbooks in Clinical Neurology. New York: Oxford University Press.

Fox, D. M., M. A. Goodale, and J. A. Bourne. 2020. The age-dependent neural substrates of blindsight. *Trends in Neurosciences* 43(4):242-252. doi: 10.1016/j.tins.2020.01.007.

Funk, C., and M. Hefferon. 2018, August 16. Most Americans accept genetic engineering of animals that benefits human health, but many oppose other uses. Pew Research Center. https://www.pewresearch.org/science/2018/08/16/most-americans-accept-genetic-engineering-of-animals-that-benefits-human-health-but-many-oppose-other-uses.

GAP (The Great Ape Project). n.d. History. https://www.projetogap.org.br/en/history.

Garrison, N. A. 2013. Genomic justice for Native Americans: Impact of the Havasupai case on genetic research. *Science, Technology, and Human Values* 38(2):201-223. doi: 10.1177/0162243912470009.

GEC (German Ethics Council). 2011. *Human-animal mixtures in research: Opinion*. Berlin: German Ethics Council. https://www.ethikrat.org/fileadmin/Publikationen/Stellungnahmen/englisch/opinion-human-animal-mixtures-in-research.pdf.

Giandomenico, S. L., S. B. Mierau, G. M. Gibbons, L. M. D. Wenger, L. Masullo, T. Sit, M. Sutcliffe, J. Boulanger, M. Tripodi, E. Derivery, O. Paulsen, A. Lakatos, and M. A. Lancaster. 2019. Cerebral organoids at the air-liquid interface generate diverse nerve tracts with functional output. *Nature Neuroscience* 22(4):669-679.

Giandomenico, S. L., M. Sutcliffe, and M. A. Lancaster. 2020. Generation and long-term culture of advanced cerebral organoids for studying later stages of neural development. *Nature Protocols*. Online ahead of print. doi: 10.1038/s41596-020-00433-w. PMID: 33328611.

Gooch, C. L., E. Pracht, and A. R. Borenstein. 2017. The burden of neurological disease in the United States: A summary report and call to action. *Annals of Neurology* 81(4):479-484. doi: 10.1002/ana.24897.

Grady, C., L. Eckstein, B. Berkman, D. Brock, R. Cook-Deegan, S. M. Fullerton, H. Greely, M. G. Hansson, S. Hull, S. Kim, B. Lo, R. Pentz, L. Rodriguez, C. Weil, B. S. Wilfond, and D. Wendler. 2015. Broad consent for research with biological samples: Workshop conclusions. *American Journal of Bioethics* 5(9):34-42. doi: 10.1080/15265161.2015.1062162.

Greely, H. T. 2020. The dilemma of human brain surrogates – Scientific opportunities, ethical concerns. In *Neuroscience and Law: Complicated Crossings and New Perspectives*, edited by Antonio D'Aloia and Maria Chiara Errigo. New York: Springer.

Greely, H. T. 2021. Human brain surrogates research: The onrushing ethical dilemma. *American Journal of Bioethics* 21(1):34-45. doi: 10.1080/15265161.2020.1845853.

Greely, H. T., and M. K. Cho. 2013. The Henrietta Lacks legacy grows. *EMBO Reports* 14(10):849. doi: 10.1038/embor.2013.148.

Greenberg, P. E., A. A. Fournier, T. Sisitsky, C. T. Pike, and R. C. Kessler. 2015. The economic burden of adults with major depressive disorder in the United States (2005 and 2010). *Journal of Clinical Psychiatry* 76(2):155-162.

Grossman, D. 2018, November 19. Scientists re-create baby brain readings in a dish. *Popular Mechanics*. https://www.popularmechanics.com/science/animals/a25224015/lab-brain-tissue-human-brain-waves.

Gruen, L. 2017. The moral status of animals. In *The Stanford Encyclopedia of Philosophy Archive*, Fall 2017 Edition, edited by Edward N. Zalta. https://plato.stanford.edu/archives/fall2017/entries/moral-animal.

Gürsoy, G., P. Emani, C. M. Brannon, O. A. Jolanki, A. Harmanci, J. S. Strattan, J. M. Cherry, A. D. Miranker, and M. Gerstein. 2020. Data sanitization to reduce private information leakage from functional genomics. *Cell* 183(4):905-917.e16. doi: 10.1016/j.cell.2020.09.036.

Han, X., M. Chen, F. Wang, M. Windrem, S. Wang, S. Shanz, Q. Xu, N. A. Oberheim, L. Bekar, S. Betstadt, A. J. Silva, T. Takano, S. A. Goldman, and M. Nedergaard. 2013. Forebrain engraftment by human glial progenitor cells enhances synaptic plasticity and learning in adult mice. *Cell Stem Cell* 12(3):342-353. doi: 10.1016/j.stem.2012.12.015.

Harriott, A. M., D. Y. Chung, A. Uner, R. O. Bozdayi, A. Morais, T. Takizawa, T. Qin, and C. Ayata. 2021. Optogenetic spreading depression elicits trigeminal pain and anxiety behavior. *Annals of Neurology* 89(1):99-110. doi: 10.1002/ana.25926.

Harward, S. C., and D. G. Southwell. 2020. Interneuron transplantation: A prospective surgical therapy for medically refractory epilepsy. *Neurosurgical Focus* 48(4):E18.

Hasselmann, J., M. A. Coburn, W. England, D. X. Figueroa Velez, S. Kiani Shabestari, C. H. Tu, A. McQuade, M. Kolahdouzan, K. Echeverria, C. Claes, T. Nakayama, R. Azevedo, N. G. Coufal, C. Z. Han, B. J. Cummings, H. Davtyan, C. K. Glass, L. M. Healy, S. P. Gandhi, R. C. Spitale, and M. Blurton-Jones. 2019. Development of a Chimeric Model to Study and Manipulate Human Microglia *In Vivo*. *Neuron* 103(6):1016-1033.e10.

Hauerwas, S. 1986. *Suffering presence: Theological Reflections on medicine, the mentally handicapped, and the church*. Notre Dame, IN: University of Notre Dame Press.

HHS (Department of Health and Human Services). 2020. *International compilation of human research standards*. https://www.hhs.gov/ohrp/international/compilation-human-research-standards/index.html.

Hodge, R. D., Bakken, T. E., J. A. Miller, K. A. Smith, E. R. Barkan, L. T. Graybuc, J. L. Close, B. Long, N. Johansen, O. Penn, Z. Yao, J. Eggermont, T. Höllt, B. Levi, S. Shehata, B. Aevermann, A. Beller, D. Bertagnolli, K. Brouner, T. Casper, C. Cobbs, R. Dalley, N. Dee, S.-L. Ding, R. Ellenbogen, O. Fong, E. Garren, J. Goldy, R. Gwinn, D. Hirschtein, D. Keene, M. Keshk, A. L. Ko, K. Lathia, A. Mahfouz, J. Maltzer, M. McGraw, T. Nguyen, J. Nyhus, J. Okjemann, A. Oldre, S. Parry, S. Reynolds, C. Rimorin, N. Shapovalova, S. Somasundaram, A. Szafer, E. Thomsen, M. Tieu, G. Quon, R. Scheuermann, R. Yuste, S. Sunkin, B. Lelieveldt, D. Feng, L. Ng, A. Bernard, M. Hawrylycz, J. Phillips, B. Tasic, H. Zeng, A. Jones, C. Koch, and E. Lein. 2019. Conserved cell types with divergent features in human versus mouse cortex. *Nature* 573(7772):61-68. doi: 10.1038/s41586-019-1506-7 PMID: 31435019.

Hu, Z., H. Li, H. Jiang, Y. Ren, X. Yu, J. Qiu, A. B. Stablewski, B. Zhang, M. J. Buck, and J. Feng. 2020. Transient inhibition of mTOR in human pluripotent stem cells enables robust formation of mouse-human chimeric embryos. *Science Advances* 6(20):eaaz0298. doi: 10.1126/sciadv.aaz0298.

Huang, Z., J. Zhang, J. Wu, G. Mashour, and A. Hudetz. 2020. Temporal circuit of macroscale dynamic brain activity supports human consciousness, *Science Advances* 6(11):eaaz0087. doi: 10.1126/sciadv.aaz0087.

Hugo, K. 2017, September 16. Exclusive: Whatever happened to the mouse with the ear on its back? *Newsweek*. https://www.newsweek.com/tissue-surgeon-ear-mouse-human-organs-transplant-cell-phones-666082.

Hunt, R. F., and S. C. Baraban. 2015. Interneuron transplantation as a treatment for epilepsy. *Cold Spring Harbor Perspectives in Medicine* 5(12):a022376. doi: 10.1101/cshperspect.a022376. PMID: 26627452.

Hyman, S. E. 2018. The daunting polygenicity of mental illness: Making a new map. *Philosophical Transactions of the Royal Society B: Biological Sciences* 373(1742):20170031. doi: 10.1098/rstb.2017.0031.

Hyun, I., J. C. Scharf-Deering, and J. E. Lunshof. 2020. Ethical issues related to brain organoid research. *Brain Research* 1732. doi: 10.1016/j.brainres.2020.146653.

IOM (Institute of Medicine). 2003. *Unequal treatment: Confronting racial and ethnic disparities in health care.* Washington, DC: The National Academies Press. doi: 10.17226/12875.

IOM. 2011. *Chimpanzees in biomedical and behavioral research: Assessing the necessity.* Washington, DC: The National Academies Press.

IPS (International Primatological Society). 2007. *International guidelines for the acquisition, care, and breeding of nonhuman primates,* 2nd ed. Captive Care Committee, International Primatological Society. http://www.internationalprimatologicalsociety.org/docs/IPS_International_Guidelines_for_the_Acquisition_Care_and_Breeding_of_Nonhuman_Primates_Second_Edition_2007. pdf.

ISSCR (International Society for Stem Cell Research). 2016. *Guidelines for Stem Cell Research and Clinical Translation.* https://www.isscr.org/policy/guidelines-for-stem-cell-research-and-clinical-translation.

Jones, H. W. Jr, V. A. McKusick, P. S. Harper, and K. D. Wuu. 1971. George Otto Gey (1899-1970): The HeLa cell and a reappraisal of its origin. *Obstetrics and Gynecology* 38(6):945-949. PMID: 4942173.

Jonsen, A. R., and S. Toulmin. 1988. *The abuse of casuistry: A history of moral reasoning.* Oakland: University of California Press. Pp. 16-20.

Ju, H., M. R. Dranias, G. Banumurthy, and A. M. VanDongen. 2015. Spatiotemporal memory is an intrinsic property of networks of dissociated cortical neurons. *Journal of Neuroscioence* 35(9):4040-4051.

Kadoshima, T., H. Sakaguchi, T. Nakano, M. Soen, S. Ando, M. Eiraku, and Y. Sasai. 2013. Self-organization of axial polarity, inside-out layer pattern, and species-specific progenitor dynamics in human ES cell-derived neocortex. *Proceedings of the National Academy of Sciences* 110(50):20284-20289.

Karzbrun, E. and O. Reiner. 2019. Brain organoids—A bottom-up approach for studying human neurodevelopment. *Bioengineering* 6(1):9 doi: 10.3390/bioengineering6010009

Kass, L. R. 1997. The wisdom of repugnance. *New Republic* 216(22).

Katsyri, J., K. Forger, M. Makarainen, and T. Takala. 2015. A review of empirical evidence on different uncanny valley hypotheses: Support for Perceptual mismatch as one road to the valley of eeriness. *Frontiers in Psychology* 6. doi: 10.3389/fpsyg.2015.00390.

Khan, T. A., O. Revah, A. Gordon, S.-J. Yoon, A. K. Krawisz, C. Goold C, Y. Sun, C. Kimg, Y. Tian, M.-Y. Li, J. Schaepe, K. Ikeda, N. Amin, N. Sakai, M. Yazawa, L. Kusha, S. Nishino, M. Porteus, J. Rapoport, J. Bernstein, R. O'Hara, C. Bearden, J. Hallmayer, J. Huguenard, D. Geschwind, R. Dolmetsch, and S. Paşca. 2018. Neuronal defects in a human cellular model of 22q11.2 deletion syndrome. *Nature Medicine* 26:1888-1898. doi: 10.1038/s41591-020-1043-9.

Kim, T. W., S. Y. Koo, and L. Studer. 2020. Pluripotent stem cell therapies for Parkinson disease: Present challenges and future opportunities. *Frontiers in Cell and Developmental Biology* 8:729. doi: 10.3389/fcell.2020.00729.

King, A. 2018, July 25. The search for better animal models of Alzheimer's disease. *Nature Outlook*. https://www.nature.com/articles/d41586-018-05722-9.

Klein, A. S., and N. Gogolla. 2021. How mice feel each other's pain or fear. *Science* 371(6525):122-123.

Knight, A. 2008. The beginning of the end for chimpanzee research? *Philosophy, Ethics, and Humanities in Medicine* 3:16. doi: 10.1186/1747-5341-3-16.

Kobayashi, T., T. Yamaguchi, S. Hamanaka, M. Kato-Itoh, Y. Yamazaki, M. Ibata, H. Sato, Y. S. Lee, J. Usui, A. S. Knisely, M. Hirabayashi, and H. Nakauchi. 2010. Generation of rat pancreas in mouse by interspecific blastocyst injection of pluripotent stem cells. *Cell* 142(5):787-799.

Koch, C., M. Massimini, M. Boly, and G. Tononi. 2016. Neural correlates of consciousness: Progress and problems. *Nature Reviews Neuroscience* 17(5):307-321.

Krienen, F., M. Goldman, Q. Zhang, R. Del Rosario, M. Florio, R. Machold, A. Saunders, K. Levandowski, H. Zaniewski, B. Schuman, C. Wu, A. Lutservitz, C. Mullally, N. Reed, E. Bien, L. Bortolin, M. Fernandez-Otero, J. Lin, A. Wysoker, J. Nemesh, D. Kulp, M. Burns, V. Tkachev, R. Smith, C. Walsh, J. Dimidschtein, B. Rudy, L. Kean, S. Berretta, G. Fishell, G. Feng, and S. McCarroll. 2020. Innovations present in the primate interneuron repertoire. *Nature* 586(7828):262-269. doi: 10.1038/s41586-020-2781-z.

Lancaster, M. A., M. Renner, C. A. Martin, D. Wenzel, L. S. Bicknell, M. E Hurles, T. Homfray, J. M. Penninger, A. P. Jackson, and J. A. Knoblich. 2013. Cerebral organoids model human brain development and microcephaly. *Nature* 501(7467):373-379.

Lassen, J. 2018. Listened to, but not heard! The failure to represent the public in genetically modified food policies. *Public Understanding of Science* 27(8). doi: 10.1177/0963662518766286.

Le Bail, R., A. Bonafina, I. Espuny-Camacho, and L. Nguyen. 2020. Learning about cell lineage, cellular diversity and evolution of the human brain through stem cell models. *Current Opinion in Neurobiology* 66:166-177.

LeDoux, J. 2012 Rethinking the emotional brain. *Neuron* 73(4):653-676.

Lee, S. S.-J., M. K. Cho, S. A. Kraft, N. Varsava, K. Gillespie, K. E. Ormond, B. S. Wilfond, and D. Magnus. 2019. "I don't want to be Henrietta Lacks": Diverse patient perspectives on donating biospecimens for precision medicine research. *Genetics in Medicine* 21:107-113. doi: 10.1038/s41436-018-0032-6.

Liao, L., L. Li, and R. C. Zhao. 2007. Stem cell research in China. *Philosophical Transactions of the Royal Society B: Biological Sciences* 362(1482):1107-1112.

Lin, C. 2020, May 16. The peril of human-animal chimera experiments. *Asia Times*.

Linaro, D., B. Vermaercke, R. Iwata, A. Ramaswamy, B. Libé-Philippot, L. Boubakar, B. A. Davis, K. Wierda, K. Davie, S. Poovathingal, P. A. Penttila, A. Bilheu, L. De Bruyne, D. Gall, K. K. Conzelmann, V. Bonin, and P. Vanderhaeghen. 2019. Xenotransplanted human cortical neurons reveal species-specific development and functional integration into mouse visual circuits. *Neuron* 104(5):972-986.

Linkenhoker, B. 2019. *Beyond IIT and GWT: Alternative empirically testable theories of consciousness.* Worldview Studio. https://1f224f96-1ca4-4a42-906d-f2724c46528f.filesusr.com/ugd/249720_e596a9e4c6be41c6885437cafc2167ae.pdf.

Loike, J. D., and M. Tendler. 2008. Reconstituting a human brain in animals: A Jewish perspective on human sanctity. *Kennedy Institute of Ethics Journal* 18(4):347-367. doi: 10.1353/ken.0.0269.

Lyn, J., J. L. Russell, D. A. Leavens, K. A. Bard, S. T. Boysen, J. A. Schaeffer, and W. D. Hopkins. 2014. Apes communicate about absent and displaced objects: Methodology matters. *Animal Cognition* 17(1):85-94. doi: 10.1007/s10071-013-0640-0.

Macintosh, K. L. 2015. Chimeras, hybrids, and cybrids: How essentialism distorts the law and stymies scientific research. *Arizona State Law Journal* 47(1).

MacLean, E. L. 2016. Unraveling the evolution of uniquely human cognition. *Proceedings of the National Academy of Sciences* 113(23):6348-6354. doi: 10.1073/pnas.1521270113.

Mansour, A. A., J. T. Gonçalves, C. W. Bloyd, H. Li, S. Fernandes, D. Quang, S. Johnston, S. L. Parylak, X. Jin, and F. H. Gage. 2018. An in vivo model of functional and vascularized human brain organoids. *Nature Biotechnology* 36(5):432-441. doi: 10.1038/nbt.4127.

Mapes, B. M., C. S. Foster, S. V. Kusnoor, M. I. Epelbaum, M. AuYoung, G. Jenkins, M. Lopez-Class, D. Richardson-Heron, A. Elmi, K. Surkan, R. M. Cronin, C. H. Wilkins, E. J. Pérez-Stable, E. Dishman, J. C. Denny, J. L. Rutter, and All of Us Research Program. 2020. Diversity and inclusion for the All of Us research program: A scoping review. *PLOS One* 15(7):e0234962. doi: 10.1371/journal.pone.0234962.

Marcus, A. D. 2018, February 23. A scientist's mission: Talking genetics with everybody. *Wall Street Journal.* https://www.wsj.com/articles/a-scientists-mission-talking-genetics-with-everybody-1519411805.

Mariani, J., G. Coppola, P. Zhang, K. Pelphery, J. Howe, and F. Vaccarino. 2015. FOXG1- dependent dysregulation of GABA/glutamate neuron differentiation in autism spectrum disorders. *Cell* 162(2):375-390. doi: 10.1016/j.cell.2015.06.034.

Masaki, H., and H. Nakauchi. 2017. Interspecies chimeras for human stem cell research. *Development* 144(14):2544-2547.

Mashour, G.A., P. Roelfsema, J. P. Changeux, and S. Dehaene. 2020. Conscious processing and the global neuronal workspace hypothesis. *Neuron* 105(5):776-798.

Mathis, A., P. Mamidanna, K. M. Cury, T. Abe, V. N. Murthy, M. W. Mathis, and M. Bethge. 2018. DeepLabCut: Markerless pose estimation of user-defined body parts with deep learning. *Nature Neuroscience* 21(9):1281-1289. doi: 10.1038/s41593-018-0209-y.

Mathis, M. W., and A. Mathis. 2020. Deep learning tools for the measurement of animal behavior in neuroscience. *Current Opinion in Neurobiology* 60:1-11. doi: 10.1016/j.conb.2019.10.008.

McLaughlin, K. 2016, March 21. China finally setting guidelines for treating lab animals. *Science.* https://www.sciencemag.org/news/2016/03/china-finally-setting-guidelines-treating-lab-animals.

Mello, M. M., and L. E. Wolf. 2010. The Havasupai Indian Tribe Case—Lessons for research involving stored biologic samples. *New England Journal of Medicine* 363:204-207. doi: 10.1056/NEJMp1005203.

Miller, G. 2012. Getting minds out of the sewer. *Science* 337(6095):679-680. doi: 10.1126/science.337.6095.679.

Miller, E. K., D. J. Freedman, and J. D. Wallis. 2002. The prefrontal cortex: Categories, concepts and cognition. *Philosophical Transactions of the Royal Society B: Biological Sciences* 357(1424):1123-1136. doi: 10.1098/rstb.2002.1099.

Miura, Y., M. Y. Li, F. Birey, K. Ikeda, O. Revah, M. V. Thete, J. Y. Park, A. Puno, S. H. Lee, M. H. Porteus, and S. P. Paşca. 2020. Generation of human striatal organoids and cortico-striatal assembloids from human pluripotent stem cells. *Nature Biotechnology* 38(12):1421-1430.

Mott, R., C. Fischer, P. Prins, and R. W. Davies. 2020. Private genomes and public SNPS: Homomorphic encryption of genotypes and phenotypes for shared quantitative genetics. *Genetics* 215(2):359-372. doi: 10.1534/genetics.120.303153.

NASEM (National Academies of Sciences, Engineering, and Medicine). 2015. *International Summit on Human Gene Editing: A global discussion*. Washington, DC: The National Academies Press. doi: 10.17226/21913.

NASEM. 2016a. *Gene drives on the horizon: Advancing science, navigating uncertainty, and aligning research with public values*. Washington, DC: The National Academies Press. doi: 10.17226/23405.

NASEM. 2016b. *Genetically engineered crops: Experiences and prospects*. Washington, DC: The National Academies Press. doi: 10.17226/23395.

NASEM. 2016c. *Mitochondrial replacement techniques: Ethical, social, and policy considerations*. Washington, DC: The National Academies Press. doi: 10.17226/21871.

NASEM. 2017a. *Human genome editing: Science, ethics, and governance*. Washington, DC: The National Academies Press. doi: 10.17226/24623. Pp. 181-194.

NASEM. 2017b. *Preparing for future products of biotechnology*. Washington, DC: The National Academies Press. doi: https://doi.org/10.17226/24605.

NASEM. 2019a. *Forest health and biotechnology: Possibilities and considerations*. Washington, DC: The National Academies Press. doi: 10.17226/25221.

NASEM. 2019b. *Second International Summit on Human Genome Editing: Continuing the global discussion: Proceedings of a workshop–in brief*. Washington, DC: The National Academies Press. doi: 10.17226/25343.

Nature Editorials. Henrietta Lacks: Science must right a historical wrong. 2020, September 1. *Nature Editorials*. doi: 10.1038/d41586-020-02494-z.

NeK. 2007. Nationale ethikkommission im Bereich Humanmedizin (2007). ethische Aspekte bei der Forschung an menschlichen embryonen und Foeten. www.nek-cne.ch

Niederauer, G. H. 2010, January 14. Free will, conscience and moral choice: What Catholics believe. Catholic News Agency. https://www.catholicnewsagency.com/column/free-will-conscience-and-moral-choice-what-catholics-believe-1087.

Niemela, J. 2011. What puts the 'yuck' in the yuck factor? *Bioethics* 25(5):267-279.

NIH (National Institutes of Health). 2009. *Guidelines for human stem cell research*. https://stemcells.nih.gov/policy/2009-guidelines.htm.

NIH. 2013. NIH to reduce significantly the use of chimpanzees in research. https://www.nih.gov/news-events/news-releases/nih-reduce-significantly-use-chimpanzees-research.

NIH. 2016. Stem cell information. stemcells.nih.gov/research/newcell_qa.htm.

NIH. 2018. U.S. Government Principles for the Utilization and Care of Vertebrate Animals Used in Testing Research and Training. Office of Laboratory Animal Welfare. https://olaw.nih.gov/policies-laws/gov-principles.htm.

NIH. 2019. Special considerations for genomics research. https://www.genome.gov/about-genomics/policy-issues/Informed-Consent-for-Genomics-Research/Special-Considerations-for-Genome-Research.

NIH. 2020. Estimates of funding for various research, condition, and disease categories (RCDC). https://report.nih.gov/categorical_spending.aspx.

Nogrady, B. 2018, July 28. These mice have brains that are part human. So are they mice, or men? *ABC Science*. https://www.abc.net.au/news/science/2018-07-29/mice-with-human-brain-cells-are-they-mice-or-men/10038550.

NRC (National Research Council). 2011. *Guide for the care and use of laboratory animals*, Eighth Edition. Washington, DC: The National Academies Press. doi: 10.17226/12910.

NRC. 2012. *International animal research regulations: Impact on neuroscience research: Workshop summary*. Washington DC: The National Academies Press. doi: 10.17226/13322.

NRC and IOM (National Research Council and Institute of Medicine). 2010. *Final report of the National Academies' Human Embryonic Stem Cell Research Advisory Committee and 2010 Amendments to the National Academies' Guidelines for Human Embryonic Stem Cell Research*. Washington, DC: The National Academies Press. doi: 10.17226/12923.

Oberheim, N., T. Takano, X. Han, W. He, J. Lin, F. Wang, Q. Xu, J. Wyatt, W. Pilcher, J. Ojemann, B. Ransom, S. Goldman, and M. Nedergaard. 2009. *Journal of Neuroscience* 29(10):3276-3287. doi: 10.1523/JNEUROSCI.4707-08.2009.

O'Doherty, K., M. M. Burgess, K. Edwards, R. P. Gallagher, A. K. Hawkins, J. Kaye, V. McCaffrey, and D. E. Winickoff. 2011. From consent to institutions: Designing adaptive governance. *Social Science and Medicine* 73(3):367-374. https://www.sciencedirect.com/science/article/pii/S0277953611003364?via%3Dihub.

Oikarinen, T., K. Srinivasan, O. Meisner, J. B. Hyman, S. Parmar, A. Fanucci-Kiss, R. Desimone, R. Landman, and G. J. Feng. 2019. Deep convolutional network for animal sound classification and source attribution using dual audio recordings. *Acoustical Society of America* 145(2):654.

OSP (Office of Science Policy). 2015. Workshop on Research with animals containing human cells. National Institutes of Health. https://osp.od.nih.gov/event/workshop-chimera/NIH.

OSP. 2016. Next steps on research using animal embryos containing human cells. National Institutes of Health. https://osp.od.nih.gov/2016/08/04/next-steps-on-research-using-animal-embryos-containing-human-cells.

Pankevich, D. E., B. M. Altevogt, J. Dunlop, F. H. Gage, and S. E. Hyman. 2014. Improving and accelerating drug development for nervous system disorders. *Neuron* 5;84(3):546-53. doi: 10.1016/j.neuron.2014.10.007.

Parker, A. 2020. The ethical cost of doing nothing. *National Science Review* 7(7):1260-1262. doi: 10.1093/nsr/nwaa095.

Paşca, S. 2018. The rise of three-dimensional human brain cultures. *Nature* 553:437-445. doi: 10.1038/nature25032.

PCB (President's Council on Bioethics). 2002. *Human cloning and human dignity: An ethical inquiry*. Washington, DC. https://bioethicsarchive.georgetown.edu/pcbe/reports/cloningreport/index.html.

PCB. 2004. *Monitoring stem cell research*. Washington, DC. https://bioethicsarchive.georgetown.edu/pcbe/reports/stemcell/index.html.

PCSBI (Presidential Commission for the Study of Bioethical Issues) 2011. *Moral science: Protecting participants in human subjects research*. https://bioethicsarchive.georgetown.edu/pcsbi/node/558.html.

PCSBI. 2015. *Gray matters: Topics at the intersection of neuroscience, ethics, and society*. https://bioethicsarchive.georgetown.edu/pcsbi/node/4704.html.

Pellegrini, L., A, Albecka, D. L. Mallery, M. J. Kellner, D. Paul, A. P. Carter, L. C. James, and M. A. Lancaster. 2020. SARS-CoV-2 infects the brain choroid plexus and disrupts the blood-CSF barrier in human brain organoids. *Cell* 27(6):951-961.e5. doi: 10.1016/j.stem.2020.10.001.

Pennartz, C. M. A., M. Farisco, and K. Evers. 2019. Indicators and criteria of consciousness in animals and intelligent machines: An inside-out approach. *Frontiers in Systems Neuroscience* 16(13):25. doi: 10.3389/fnsys.2019.00025.

Piotrowska, M. 2020. Rethinking the oversight conditions of human–animal chimera research. *Bioethics* 35(1):98-104. doi: 10.1111/bioe.12797.

Popejoy, A. B., and S. M. Fullerton. 2016. Genomics is failing on diversity. *Nature* 538(7624):161-164. doi: 10.1038/538161a.

Qian, X., H. N. Nguyen, F. Jacob, H. Song, G. L. Ming. 2017. Using brain organoids to understand Zika virus-induced microcephaly. *Development* 144(6):952-957.

Qiu, P., J. Jiang, Z. Liu, Y. Cai, T. Huang, Y. Wang, Q. Liu, Y. Nie, F. Liu, J. Cheng, Q. Li, Y.- C. Tang, M. Poo, Z. Sun, and H.-C. Chiang. 2019. BMAL1 knockout macaque monkeys display reduced sleep and psychiatric disorders. *National Science Review* 6(1):87-100. doi: 10.1093/nsr/nwz002.

Quadrato, G., J. Brown, and P. Arlotta. 2016. The promises and challenges of human brain organoids as models of neuropsychiatric disease. *Nature Medicine* 22(11):1220-1228.

Quadrato, G., T. Nguyen, E. Z. Macosko, J. L. Sherwood, S. Min Yang, D. R. Berger, N. Maria, J. Scholvin, M. Goldman, J. P. Kinney, E. Boyden, J. Lichtman, Z. Williams, S. McCarroll, and O. Arlotta. 2017. Cell diversity and network dynamics in photosensitive human brain organoids. *Nature* 545(7652):48-53.

REFERENCES

Ram, N., C. J. Guerrini, and A. L. McGuire. 2018. Genealogy databases and the future of criminal investigation. *Science* 360(6393):1078-1079. doi: 10.1126/science.aau1083.

Rao, R. 2016. Informed consent, body property, and self-sovereignty. *Journal of Law, Medicine, and Ethics* 44(3). doi: 10.1177/1073110516667940.

Rayon, T., D. Stamataki, R. Perez-Carrasco, L. Garcia-Perez, C. Barrington, M. Melchionda, K. Exelby, J. Lazaro, V. L. J. Tybulewicz, E. M. C. Fisher, and J. Briscoe. 2020. Species-specific pace of development is associated with differences in protein stability. *Science* 369(6510):eaba7667.

Regalado, A. 2019, August 1. Scientists are making human-monkey hybrids in China. *MIT Technology Review*. https://www.technologyreview.com/2019/08/01/652/scientists-are-making-human-monkey-hybrids-in-china.

Rifes, P., M. Isaksson, G. S. Rathore, P. Aldrin-Kirk, O. K. Møller, G. Barzaghi, J. Lee, K. L. Egerod, D. M. Rausch, M. Parmar, T. Pers, T. Laurell, and A. Kirkeby. 2020. Modeling neural tube development by differentiation of human embryonic stem cells in a microfluidic WNT gradient. *Nature Biotechnology* 38:1265-1273.

Robert, J. S., and F. Baylis. 2003. Crossing species boundaries. *American Journal of Bioethics* 3(3):1-13. doi: 10.1162/15265160360706417.

Rozin, P. 2015. Disgust, psychology of. In *International Encyclopedia of the Social & Behavioral Sciences*, 2nd edition, Vol. 6, edited by J. D. Wright. Oxford: Elsevier. Pp. 546-549.

Rozin, P., and J. Haidt. 2013. The domains of disgust and their origins: Contrasting biological and cultural evolutionary accounts. *Trends in Cognitive Sciences* 17(8):367-368. doi: 10.1016/j.tics.2013.06.001.

Sanes, J. R. 2021. Experience and refinement of synaptic connections. In *Principles of Neural Science*, 6th edition. Edited by E. R. Kandel, T. M. Jessll, S. A. Seigelbaum, S. H. Mack, and J. B. Koester. New York: McGraw Hill. Pp. 1200-1225.

Sato, T., R. G. Vries, H. J. Snippert, M. van de Wetering, N. Barker, D. E. Stange, J. H. van Es, A. Abo, P. Kujala, P. J. Peters, and H. Clevers. 2009. Single Lgr5 stem cells build crypt-villus structures in vitro without a mesenchymal niche. *Nature* 459(7244):262-265.

Scheufele, D. A., N. M. Krause, I. Freiling, and D. Brossard. 2021. What we know about effective public engagement on CRISPR and beyond. *Proceedings of the National Academy of Sciences of the United States of America*. DOI: 10.1073/pnas.2004835117.

Schmidt, C. W. 2008. The yuck factor when disgust meets discovery. *Environmental Health Perspectives* 116(12).

Schuster, B., M. Junkin, S. S. Kashaf, I. Romero-Calvo, K. Kirby, J. Matthews, C. R. Weber, A. Rzhetsky, K. P. White, and S. Tay. 2020. Automated microfluidic platform for dynamic and combinatorial drug screening of tumor organoids. *Nature Communications* 11(1):5271.

Scott, A. W., N. M. Bressler, S. Ffolkes, J. S. Wittenborn, and J. Jorkasky. 2016. Public attitudes about eye and vision health. *JAMA Ophthalmology* 134(10):1111-1118. doi: 10.1001/jamaophthalmol.2016.2627.

Scott, S. E., Y. Inbar, C. D. Wirz, D. Brossard, and P. Rozin P. 2018. An overview of attitudes toward genetically engineered food. *Annual Review of Nutrition* 38:459-479. doi: 10.1146/annurev-nutr-071715-051223.

Seth, A. K., B. J. Baars, and D. B. Edelman. 2005. Criteria for consciousness in humans and other mammals. *Consciousness and Cognition* 14(1):119-139. doi: 10.1016/j.concog.2004.08.006.

Shah, N. R. 2013. NYSTEM: Igniting a thriving stem cell research community. *STEM CELLS Translational Medicine* 2(5):325-327. doi: 10.5966/sctm.2013-0057.

Shaw, D. 2014. Creating chimeras for organs is legal in Switzerland. *Bioethics Forum* 7(24).

Sierksma, A., V. Escott-Price, and B. De Strooper. 2020. Translating genetic risk of Alzheimer's disease into mechanistic insight and drug targets. *Science* 70(6512):61-66.

Skloot, R. 2010. *The Immortal Life of Henrietta Lacks*. New York: Crown.

Sladek, J. R. Jr., and D. M. Gash. 1988. Nerve-cell grafting in Parkinson's disease. *Journal of Neurosurgery* 68(3):337-351.

Smith, J. D. 2010. Inaugurating the study of animal metacognition. *International Journal of Comparative Psychology* 23(3):401-413.

Smith, W. J. 2020, October 29. Will scientists create a conscious human brain in a dish? *National Review*. https://www.nationalreview.com/corner/will-scientists-create-a-conscious-human-brain-in-a-dish.

Smits, M. 2006. Taming monsters: The cultural domestication of new technology. *Technology in Society* 28(4):489-504. doi: 10.1016/j.techsoc.2006.09.008.

Sood, D., M. Tang-Schomer, D. Pouli, C. Mizzoni, N. Raia, A. Tai, K. Arkun, J. Wu, L. D. Black 3rd, B. Scheffler, I. Georgakoudi, D. Steindler, and D. Kaplan. 2019. 3D extracellular matrix microenvironment in bioengineered tissue models of primary pediatric and adult brain tumors. *Nature Communications* 10:4529.

Southwell, D. G., C. R. Nicholas, A. I. Basbaum, M. P. Stryker, A. R. Kriegstein, J. L. Rubenstein, and A. Alvarez-Buylla. 2014. Interneurons from embryonic development to cell-based therapy. *Science* 344(6180):1240622.

Staley K., and D. Barron. 2019. Learning as an outcome of involvement in research: what are the implications for practice, reporting and evaluation? *Research Involvement and Engagement* 5(14). doi:10.1186/s40900-019-0147-1.

Stetka, B. 2019, August 29. Lab-grown 'mini brains' can now mimic the neural activity of a preterm infant. *Scientific American*. https://www.scientificamerican.com/article/lab-grown-mini-brains-can-now-mimic-the-neural-activity-of-a-preterm-infant.

Streiffer, R. 2008. Informed consent and federal funding for stem cell research. *Hastings Center Report* 38(3):40-47.

Streiffer, R. 2019. Human/non-human chimeras. In *The Stanford Encyclopedia of Philosophy Archive*, edited by Edward N. Zalta. https://plato.stanford.edu/entries/chimeras.

Sugarman, J., and A. Bredenoord. 2019. Q&A: Reflections on organoid ethics. *Cell Stem Cell* 24(6):849-851. doi: 10.1016/j.stem.2019.05.010.

Sun, L., R. Liu, F. Guo, M. Q. Wen, X. L. Ma, K. Y. Li, H. Sun, C. L. Xu, Y. Y. Li, M. Y. Wu, Z. G. Zhu, X. J. Li, Y. Q. Yu, Z. Chen, X. Y. Li, and S. Duan. 2020. Parabrachial nucleus circuit governs neuropathic pain-like behavior. *Nature Communications* 11(1):5974.

Swiss Academy of Medical Sciences. 2009. *Interspecies crosses: Aspects of animal protection*. Ethics Committee for Animal Studies of the Swiss Academy of Medical Sciences and Swiss Academy of Sciences. https://www.altex.org/index.php/altex/article/view/612/620.

Takahashi, K., and S. Yamanaka. 2006. Induction of pluripotent stem cells from mouse embryonic and adult fibroblast cultures by defined factors. *Cell* 126(4):663-676.

Tlili, S. 2018. Animal ethics in Islam. *Religions* 9(9):269. https://doi.org/10.3390/rel9090269.

Tomasello, M., and J. Call. 2019. Thirty years of great ape gestures. *Animal Cognition* 22(4):461-469. doi: 10.1007/s10071-018-1167-1.

Tononi, G., M. Boly, M. Massimini, and C. Koch. 2016. Integrated information theory: From consciousness to its physical substrate. *Nature Reviews Neuroscience* 17:450-461. doi: 10.1038/nrn.2016.44.

Trautmann, S., J. Rehm, and H. U. Wittchen. 2016. Psychiatric disease burden: The economic costs of mental disorders: Do our societies react appropriately to the burden of mental disorders? *EMBO Reports* 17(9):1245-1249. PMID: 27491723.

Trujillo, C. A., R. Gao, P. D. Negraes, G. W. Yeo, B. Voytek, and A. R. Muotri. 2019. Complex oscillatory waves emerging from cortical organoids model early human brain network development. *Cell Stem Cell* 25(4):558-569.e7. doi: 10.1016/j.stem.2019.08.002.

Twitty, V. C. 1937. Experiments on the phenomenon of paralysis produced by a toxin occurring in Triturus embryos. *Journal of Experimental Zoology* 76:67-104.

Ueno, M., M. Matsumura, K. Watanabe, T. Nakamura, F. Osakada, M. Takahashi, H. Kawasaki, S. Kinoshita, and Y. Sasai. 2006. Neural conversion of ES cells by an inductive activity on human amniotic membrane matrix. *Proceedings of the National Academy of Sciences* 103(25):9554-9559. doi: 10.1073/pnas.0600104103.

Upadhya, D., B. Hattiangady, O. W. Castro, B. Shuai, M. Kodali, S. Attaluri, A. Bates, Y. Dong, C. Zhang, D. J. Prockop, and A. K. Shetty. 2019. Human induced pluripotent stem cell-derived MGE cell grafting after status epilepticus attenuates chronic epilepsy and comorbidities via synaptic integration. *Proceedings of the National Academy of Sciences* 116(1):287-296.

Uzel, S. G., O. C. Amadi, T. M. Pearl, R. T. Lee, P. T. So, and R. D. Kamm. 2016. Simultaneous or sequential orthogonal gradient formation in a 3D cell culture microfluidic platform. *Small* 12: 612-622.

Van Gulick, R. 2018. Consciousness. In *The Stanford Encyclopedia of Philosophy Archive*, edited by Edward N. Zalta. https://plato.stanford.edu/entries/consciousness.

Vanderbilt University Medical Center. 2015, January 29. Consent process for BioVU participation updated. https://news.vumc.org/2015/01/29/consent-process-for-biovu-participation-updated.

Velasco, S., A. J. Kedaigle, S. K. Simmons, A. Nash, M. Rocha, G. Quadrato, B. Paulsen, L. Nguyen, X. Adiconis, A. Regev, J. Z. Levin, and P. Arlotta. 2019. Individual brain organoids reproducibly form cell diversity of the human cerebral cortex. *Nature* 570(7762):523-527.

Velasco, S., B. Paulsen, and P. Arlotta. 2020. 3D brain organoids: Studying brain development and disease outside the embryo. *Annual Review of Neuroscience* 43:375-389.

Verhey, A. 1995. "Playing God" and invoking a perspective. *Journal of Medicine and Philosophy* 20(4):347-364. doi: 10.1093/jmp/20.4.347.

Watanabe, K., M. Ueno, D. Kamiya, A. Nishiyama, M. Matsumura, T. Wataya, J. Takahashi, S. Nishikawa, S. Mishikawa, K. Muguruma, and Y. Sasai. 2007. A ROCK inhibitor permits survival of dissociated human embryonic stem cells. *Nature Biotechnology* 25(6):681-686.

Weatherall, D. 2006. *The use of non-human primates in research: A working group report*. FRS FMedSci. https://mrc.ukri.org/documents/pdf/the-use-of-non-human-primates-in-research.

The Week. Should apes have legal rights? 2013, August 13. *The Week*. https://theweek.com/articles/461480/should-apes-have-legal-rights.

Wiltschko, A. B., T. Tsukahara, A. Zeine, R. Anyoha, W. F. Gillis, J. E. Markowitz, R. E. Peterson, J. Katon, M. J. Johnson, and S. R. Datta. 2020. Revealing the structure of pharmacobehavioral space through motion sequencing. *Nature Neuroscience* 23(11):1433-1443.

Windrem, M. S., S. J. Schanz, L. Zou, D. Chandler-Militello, N. J. Kuypers, M. Nedergaard, Y. Lu, J. N. Mariani, and S. A. Goldman. 2020. Human glial progenitor cells effectively remyelinate the demyelinated adult brain. *Cell Reports* 31(7):107658.

Wise, S. P. 2008. Forward frontal fields: Phylogeny and fundamental function. *Trends in Neuroscience* 31:599-608.

Wolinetz, C. D., and F. S. Collins. 2020. Recognition of research participants' need for autonomy: Remembering the legacy of Henrietta Lacks. *Journal of the American Medical Association* 324(11):1027-1028. doi: 10.1001/jama.2020.15936.

World Medical Association. 1964. *Declaration of Helsinki—Ethical principles for medical research involving human subjects*. https://www.wma.net/policies-post/wma-declaration-of-helsinki-ethical-principles-for-medical-research-involving-human-subjects.

Wu, J., A. Platero-Luengo, M. Sakurai, A. Sugawara, M. A. Gil, T, Yamauchi, K. Suzuki, Y. Bogliotti, C. Cuello, M. Morales Valencia, D. Okumura, J. Luo, M. Vilariño, I. Parrilla, D. Soto, C. Martinez, T. Hishida, S. Sánchez-Bautista, M. L. Martinez-Martinez, H. Wang, A. Nohalez, E. Aizawa, P. Martinez-Redondo, A. Ocampo, P. Reddy, J. Roca, E. Maga, C. Rodriguez Esteban, W. T. Berggren, E. Nuñez Delicado, J. Lajara, I. Guillen, P. Guillen, J. Campistol, E. Martinez, P. Ross, and J. Izpisua Belmonte. 2017. Interspecies chimerism with mammalian pluripotent stem cells. *Cell* 168(3):473-486.e15.

Xiong, M., Y. Tao, Q. Gao, B. Feng, W. Yan, Y. Zhou, T. A. Kotsonis, T. Yuan, Z. You, Z. Wu, J. Xi, A. Haberman, J. Graham, J. Block, W. Zhou, Y. Chen, and S. C. Zhang. 2021. Human stem cell-derived neurons repair circuits and restore neural function. *Cell Stem Cell* 28(1):112-126.e6.

Ye, F., E. Kang, C. Yu, X. Qian, F. Jacob, C. Yu, M. Mao, R. Poon, J. Kim, H. Song, G.-L. Ming, and M. Zhang. 2017. DISC1 regulates neurogenesis via modulating kinetochore attachment of Ndel1/Nde1 during mitosis. *Neuron* 96:1041-1054.

Yoon, S.-J., L. S. Elahi, A. M. Paşca, R. M. Marton, A. Gordon, O. Revah, Y. Miura, E. M. Walczak, G. M. Holdgate, H. C. Fan, J. R. Huguenard, D. H. Geschwind, and S. P. Paşca. 2019. Reliability of human cortical organoid generation. *Nature Methods* 16:75-78.

Young, R. 2020. Voluntary euthanasia. In *The Stanford Encyclopedia of Philosophy Archive*, edited by Edward N. Zalta. https://plato.stanford.edu/archives/spr2020/entries/euthanasia-voluntary.

Zhang, S. C., M. Wernig, I. D. Duncan, O. Brüstle, and J. A. Thomson. 2001. In vitro differentiation of transplantable neural precursors from human embryonic stem cells. *Nature Biotechnology* 19(12):1129-1133.

Zhou, Y., J. Sharma, Q. Ke, R. Landman, J. Yuan, H. Chen, D. S. Hayden, J. W. Fisher 3rd, M. Jiang, W. Menegas, T. Aida, T. Yan, Y. Zou, D. Xu, S. Parmar, J. B. Hyman, A. Fanucci-Kiss, O. Meisner, D. Wang, Y. Huang, Y. Li, Y. Bai, W. Ji, X. Lai, W. Li, L. Huang, Z. Lu, L. Wang, S. A. Anteraper, M. Sur, H. Zhou, A. P. Xiang, R. Desimone, G. Feng, and S. Yang. 2019. Atypical behaviour and connectivity in SHANK3-mutant macaques. *Nature* 570(7761):326-331.

Zimmer, K. 2019, April 4. Bioethicists concerned over Japan's chimera embryo regulations. *The Scientist*. https://www.the-scientist.com/news-opinion/bioethicists-concerned-over-japans-chimera-embryo-regulations-65700.

Zirui, H., J. Zhang, J. Wu, G. A. Mashour, and A. G. Hudetz. 2020. Temporal circuit of macroscale dynamic brain activity supports human consciousness. *Science Advances* 6(11):eaaz0087. doi: 10.1126/sciadv.aaz0087.

Appendix A

Biographies of Committee and Staff Members

Co-Chairs

Bernard Lo, M.D., is professor emeritus of medicine and director emeritus of the Program in Medical Ethics at the University of California, San Francisco (UCSF) and president emeritus of the Greenwall Foundation. A member of the National Academy of Medicine (NAM), Dr. Lo has chaired NAM committees on Sharing Clinical Trial Data (2015); Conflict of Interest in Medical Research, Education, and Practice (2009); and Evidence-based Clinical Practice Guidelines for Prescribing Opioids for Acute Pain (2019). He currently serves on the California COVID-19 Vaccine Drafting Guidelines Workgroup and on the California Health Care Surge & Crisis Care Guidelines Advisory Group. Dr. Lo also chairs the external advisory board of the Multiregional Clinical Trials Network and serves on the Medical Advisory Panel of Blue Cross/Blue Shield and the Ethics Advisory Council for Takeda Pharmaceuticals. He and his colleagues have published over 200 peer-reviewed articles on ethical issues concerning decision making near the end of life, the doctor–patient relationship, responsible oversight of research, and conflicts of interest. During the COVID-19 pandemic Dr. Lo and his colleagues have written articles on cardiopulmonary resuscitation, addressing vaccine hesitancy, and allocation of ventilators and inpatient medications. He is the author of *Resolving Ethical Dilemmas: A Guide for Clinicians* (6th ed., 2019). Dr. Lo continues to care for a panel of primary care internal medicine patients at UCSF.

Joshua R. Sanes, Ph.D., is Jeff C. Tarr professor of molecular and cellular biology and Paul J. Finnegan family director of the Center for Brain Science at Harvard University. Dr. Sanes uses molecular, genetic, and imaging approaches to understand how synapses form, mature, and function. The Center he directs supports an interdisciplinary approach that combines biology, chemistry, engineering, and psychology to look at circuit-level questions in neuroscience. Dr. Sanes also served for more than 20 years on the faculty of Washington University in St. Louis, where he held an endowed chair. He has authored over 300 publications and is a highly sought-after presenter at national and international symposia. Dr. Sanes is a member of the National Academy of Sciences, a fellow of the American Association for the Advancement of Science and the American Academy of Arts and Sciences, and a recipient of the Alden Spencer Award of Columbia University. He has served on the National Advisory Council of the National Institute of Neurological Disorders and Stroke, the Council of the Society for Neuroscience, and advisory panels for the Muscular Dystrophy Association, the Amyotrophic Lateral Sclerosis (ALS) Association, the Klingenstein Neuroscience Fund, the Searle Scholars Fund, the Stowers Institute for Medical Research, and the Howard Hughes Medical Institute. After graduating from Yale University in 1970 with degrees in biochemistry and psychology, Dr. Sanes earned a Ph.D. in neurobiology from Harvard in 1976. He completed postdoctoral work at the University of California, San Francisco.

Members

Paola Arlotta, Ph.D., is chair and Golub Family professor of the Department of Stem Cell and Regenerative Biology and a college professor at Harvard University. She is also an associate member of the Stanley Center for Psychiatric Research at the Broad Institute of the Massachusetts Institute of Technology and Harvard University. Collectively, the Arlotta Lab research program explores the interface between development and engineering of the neocortex to gain fundamental understanding of both the principles that govern normal cortical development and of previously inaccessible mechanisms of human neurodevelopmental disease. The lab aims to understand and model complex human cortical pathology, focusing on the development of new high-throughput in vitro models of human cortical development and neurodevelopmental disease using stem cell–derived 3D brain organoids. Dr. Arlotta is the recipient of many awards, including the 2017 George Ledlie Prize from Harvard, the Fannie Cox Prize for Excellence in Science Teaching, the 2018 Friedrich Wilhelm Bessel Research Award from the Humboldt Foundation, and a 2019 Harvard College Professorship. Dr. Arlotta received an M.S. in biochemistry from the University of Trieste, Italy, and a Ph.D. in molecular biology from the University of Portsmouth, UK. She subsequently completed her postdoctoral training in neuroscience at Harvard Medical School.

Alta Charo, J.D., is Knowles professor emerita of law and bioethics at the University of Wisconsin–Madison (UW) and David A. Hamburg distinguished fellow at the Nuclear Threat Initiative, where she is a member of the Biosecurity Innovation and Risk Reduction Initiative. At UW she taught bioethics, biotechnology regulation and policy, and public health law and torts until 2020. Prior to her arrival at UW in 1989, Ms. Charo served as associate director of the Legislative Drafting Research Fund of Columbia University, Fulbright lecturer in American law at the Sorbonne in Paris, legal analyst at the congressional Office of Technology Assessment, and American Association for the Advancement of Science (AAAS) diplomacy fellow at USAID. Also in government, she was a member of President Clinton's National Bioethics Advisory Commission and a policy advisor in the Food and Drug Administration's Office of the Commissioner. At the National Academies of Sciences, Engineering, and Medicine, Ms. Charo has served on numerous committees, including the Committee on Science, Technology, and Law; the committee that issued the 2004 report *Biotechnology Research in the Age of Terrorism*; and committees on emerging infectious diseases and COVID-19 vaccine and monoclonal antibody allocation frameworks. She co-chaired the National Academies committees that wrote guidelines for embryonic stem cell research and developed recommendations for U.S. policy and global principles for human genome editing research and clinical trials. Ms. Charo now co-chairs the National Academy of Medicine (NAM) Committee on Emerging Science, Technology, and Innovation and serves on the World Health Organization's committee on global governance of genome editing. She is a member of the NAM and an elected Fellow of the AAAS and of the American Academy of Arts and Sciences.

John H. Evans, Ph.D., is Tata Chancellor's endowed professor in social sciences, associate dean of social sciences, and codirector of the Institute for Practical Ethics at the University of California, San Diego (UCSD). He has been a visiting member at the Institute for Advanced Study and a postdoctoral fellow at Yale University, and he has held visiting professorial fellowships or honorary professorships at the Universities of Edinburgh, Muenster, Ben Gurion, and Queensland. Originally trained as a sociologist of religion, Dr. Evans has focused on the abstract human concerns often addressed by Western religions such as the nature of the human, intergenerational responsibility, and societal value pluralism. More specifically, his research focuses on politics, religion, science, and ethics, with a particular interest in examining humanistic questions using quantitative and qualitative social science methodologies. Dr. Evans has published seven books and over 50 articles and volume chapters. From 2015 to 2017, he was a member of the National Academies of Sciences, Engineering, and Medicine Committee on Human Gene Editing: Scientific, Medical and Ethical Considerations. Dr. Evans earned a B.A. from Macalester College and a Ph.D. from Princeton University.

Fred H. Gage, Ph.D., is president and professor at the Laboratory of Genetics and Vi and John Adler chair for research on age-related neurodegenerative disease at the Salk Institute for Biological Studies in La Jolla, California. He is also past president of the Society for Neuroscience and the International Society for Stem Cell Research. Dr. Gage's research is concentrated on the unexpected plasticity and adaptability to the environment that mammals exhibit throughout life. His lab showed that human beings and other mammals are capable of growing new nerve cells throughout life, in a process called adult neurogenesis. Dr. Gage's team explores how these cells can be prompted to become mature, functioning nerve cells in the adult brain and spinal cord. He has also shown that environmental enrichment and physical exercise can enhance the growth of new brain cells, and his team continues to study the underlying cellular and molecular mechanisms of neurogenesis to find possible avenues to repair damaged or aging brains. Dr. Gage's lab also models diseases in the laboratory using human stem cells, seeking to decipher the progression and mechanisms that lead to brain cell dysfunction. He is a member of the American Academy of Arts and Sciences, EMBO, and the American Philosophical Society. Dr. Gage earned a B.S. from the University of Florida, and both an M.S. and Ph.D. from The Johns Hopkins University.

Henry T. "Hank" Greely, J.D., is Deane F. and Kate Edelman Johnson professor of law and professor, by courtesy, of genetics at Stanford University, where he has been teaching since 1985. He specializes in ethical, legal, and social issues arising from advances in the biosciences, particularly from genetics, neuroscience, and human stem cell research. Professor Greely directs the Stanford Center for Law and the Biosciences, chairs the California Advisory Committee on Human Stem Cell Research, and serves on the Neuroscience Forum of the National Academy of Medicine. From 2007 to 2010 he was a codirector of the Law and Neuroscience Project, and in 2006, he was elected a fellow of the American Association for Advancement of Science.

Professor Greely served as a law clerk for Judge John Minor Wisdom on the U.S. Court of Appeals and for Justice Potter Stewart of the U.S. Supreme Court. After working during the Carter administration in the Departments of Defense and Energy, he entered private practice in Los Angeles in 1981 as a litigator with the law firm of Tuttle & Taylor, Inc. Professor Greely graduated from Stanford University in 1974 and from Yale Law School in 1977.

Patricia A. King, J.D., is professor emerita of law at Georgetown University Law Center and adjunct professor in the Department of Health Policy and Management in the Johns Hopkins Bloomberg School of Public Health. With expertise in the study of law, medicine, ethics, and public policy, she teaches family law courses and a seminar in bioethics and the law, and is coauthor of *Cases and Materials on Law, Science and Medicine*. Professor King is a member of the American Law Institute and the National Academy of Medicine, and is a fellow of the Hastings Center. Her work in the field of bioethics has included service on the National Institutes of Health Recombinant DNA Advisory Committee; the President's Commission for the Study of Ethical Problems in Medicine and Biomedical and Behavioral Research; the National Commission for the Protection of Human Subjects of Biomedical and Behavioral Research; and the Ethics, Legal and Social Issues Working Group of the Human Genome Project. Professor King is a fellow of the Harvard Corporation and a member of the board of trustees of Wheaton College. Her professional experience before joining the Law Center faculty in 1973 was primarily in the field of civil rights; she was the deputy director of the Office of Civil Rights and special assistant to the chairman of the U.S. Equal Employment Opportunity Commission, and she served as a deputy assistant attorney general in the Civil Division of the Department of Justice. Professor King earned a B.A. from Wheaton College and a J.D. from Harvard Law School.

William T. "Bill" Newsome, Ph.D., is Harman Family Provostial professor of neurobiology at the Stanford University School of Medicine and Vincent V.C. Woo director of the Wu Tsai Neurosciences Institute. A leading investigator in systems and cognitive neuroscience, he has made fundamental contributions to our understanding of the neural mechanisms underlying visual perception and simple forms of decision making. Among Dr. Newsome's honors are the Rank Prize in Optoelectronics, the Spencer Award, the Distinguished Scientific Contribution Award of the American Psychological Association, the Dan David Prize of Tel Aviv University, the Karl Spencer Lashley Award of the American Philosophical Society, and the Champalimaud Vision Award. His distinguished lectureships include the 13th Annual Marr Lecture at the University of Cambridge, the 9th Annual Brenda Milner Lecture at McGill University, and most recently, the Distinguished Visiting Scholar Lectures at the Kavli Institute of Brain and Mind at the University of California, San Diego. Dr. Newsome was elected to membership in the National Academy of Sciences in 2000 and to the American Philosophical Society in 2011. He co-chaired the National Institutes of Health BRAIN Working Group, charged with forming a national plan for the coming decade of neuroscience research in the United States. Dr. Newsome received a B.S. in physics from Stetson University and a Ph.D. in biology from the California Institute of Technology.

Sally Temple, Ph.D., is scientific director of the Neural Stem Cell Institute and oversees scientific programs with the goal of understanding the role of neural stem cells in central nervous system (CNS) development, maintenance, and repair. She is past member of the board of directors and president of the International Society for Stem Cell Research. Dr. Temple leads a team of 30 researchers focused on using neural stem cells to develop therapies for eye, brain, and spinal cord disorders. In 2008, she was awarded the MacArthur Fellowship Award for her contribution and future potential in the neural stem cell field. In 1989, Dr. Temple discovered that the embryonic mammalian brain contained a rare stem cell that could be activated to proliferate in vitro and produce both neurons and glia. Since then, her lab has continued to make pioneering contributions to the field of stem cell research by characterizing neural stem cells and the intrinsic and environmental factors that regulate their behavior. Dr. Temple helps lead the Tau Consortium, an international, collaborative group focused on understanding and developing therapies for dementias. Dr. Temple received an undergraduate degree from Cambridge University, specializing in developmental biology and neuroscience. She performed her Ph.D. work in optic nerve development at University College London in the United Kingdom. She received a Royal Society Fellowship to support her postdoctoral work at Columbia University, NY, where she focused on spinal cord development.

Lawrence "Larry" Zipursky, Ph.D., is Jerome J. Belzer chair of medical research and distinguished professor of biological chemistry at University of California, Los Angeles (UCLA) and an investigator of the Howard Hughes Medical Institute. He studies brain development, focusing on how neural circuits are formed during development, and his laboratory has provided insights into various aspects of circuit assembly, including the molecular basis of neuronal identity through their work on the Dscam1 locus in Drosophila. Dr. Zipursky was elected fellow of the American Academy of Arts and Sciences in 1998 and a member of the National Academy of Sciences in 2009. He received the Louisa Gross Horwitz Prize for Biology and Biochemistry from Columbia University in 2015. In 1981, Dr. Zipursky moved to the California Institute of Technology as a Helen Hay Whitney postdoctoral fellow. He has served on the National Advisory Council of the National Institute of Neurological Disorders and Stroke and various scientific advisory panels including the McKnight, the Helen Hay Whitney, and the Alfred P. Sloan foundations. Dr. Zipursky received a Ph.D. in molecular biology at Albert Einstein College of Medicine, where he completed his thesis with Dr. Jerard Hurwitz, studying DNA replication in E. coli.

Staff

Anne-Marie Mazza, Ph.D., senior director, joined the National Academies of Sciences, Engineering, and Medicine in 1995 as a program officer with the Government-University-Industry Research Roundtable, and in 1999 co-launched the Committee on Science, Technology, and Law (CSTL). She has led numerous National Academies consensus studies including *Securing the Vote: Protecting American Democracy, Dual Use Research of Concern in the Life Sciences, Optimizing the Nation's Investment in Academic Research, Identifying the Culprit: Assessing Eyewitness Identification, Strengthening Forensic Science in the United States, Science and Security in A Post 9/11 World*, and the 3rd edition of the *Reference Manual on Scientific Evidence*. Dr. Mazza was staff director for the 2015 and 2018 International Summits on Human Genome Editing and the 2020

National Academy of Sciences symposium *Science: The Endless Frontier*. From 1999 to 2000, she was a senior policy analyst with the White House Office of Science and Technology Policy where she directed a presidential review of the government–university research partnership. Dr. Mazza directed the National Academies' Christine Mirzayan Science and Technology Policy Graduate Fellowship Program from 2007 to 2018 and served as senior director of strategic initiatives in the National Academy of Medicine President's Office from 2018 to 2019. Currently, she is senior director of CSTL; the Committee on Science, Engineering, Medicine, and Public Policy; and the National Science, Technology, and Security Roundtable. She is senior leader of the U.S. Science and Innovation Policy Portfolio and a fellow of the American Association for the Advancement of Science. Dr. Mazza received a B.A., M.A., and Ph.D., from The George Washington University.

Steven Kendall, Ph.D., is a program officer for the Committee on Science, Technology, and Law at the National Academies of Sciences, Engineering, and Medicine. He has contributed to numerous National Academies reports, including *Securing the Vote: Protecting American Democracy* (2018); *Optimizing the Nation's Investment in Academic Research* (2016); *International Summit on Human Gene Editing: A Global Discussion* (2015); *Identifying the Culprit: Assessing Eyewitness Identification* (2014); *Positioning Synthetic Biology to Meet the Challenges of the 21st Century* (2013); the *Reference Manual on Scientific Evidence*, 3rd Edition (2011); *Review of the Scientific Approaches Used During the FBI's Investigation of the 2001 Anthrax Mailings* (2011); *Managing University Intellectual Property in the Public Interest* (2010); and *Strengthening Forensic Science in the United States: A Path Forward* (2009). Prior to joining the National Academies in 2007, Dr. Kendall worked at the Smithsonian American Art Museum and The Huntington in San Marino, California. He received an M.A. in Victorian art and architecture at the University of London and completed a Ph.D. in the Department of the History of Art and Architecture at the University of California, Santa Barbara.

Anita Eisenstadt, J.D., is a program officer in the U.S. Science and Innovation Policy Theme of the National Academies of Sciences, Engineering, and Medicine. She previously served as assistant vice president for research integrity at Oregon State University, where she oversaw university compliance with federal research regulations. Ms. Eisenstadt previously served as a senior foreign affairs officer for Europe and the Organisation for Economic Co-operation and Development (OECD) in the State Department's Office of Science and Technology Cooperation. At the State Department, she formulated U.S. foreign policy on science, technology, and innovation and led U.S. delegations to the OECD Committee on Science and Technology Policy and its Working Party on Biotechnology. Prior to joining the State Department, Ms. Eisenstadt served as assistant general counsel at the National Science Foundation (NSF). She served as NSF's lead attorney on international, Antarctic, legislative, environmental, information policy, and research compliance matters, and she established a Special Deputy U.S. Marshal Program in Antarctica and co-drafted the federal research misconduct policy. At NSF, Ms. Eisenstadt also served on U.S. delegations to the United Nations International Maritime Organization, the United Nations World Summit on the Information Society, the Antarctic Treaty System, and the Legal Experts' Group developing an Antarctic environmental liability regime. She earned a B.A. in anthropology and Asian studies from the University of Michigan and a J.D. from Wayne State University Law School.

Vernon "Vern" Dunn, Ph.D., is a program officer in the U.S. Science and Innovation Policy Theme of the National Academies of Sciences, Engineering, and Medicine. Since joining the National Academies in early 2020, his role has included work with the Committee on Science, Engineering, Medicine, and Public Policy; the Committee on Science, Technology, and Law; and the New Voices in Sciences, Engineering, and Medicine program. Prior to joining the National Academies, Dr. Dunn worked with a small firm in Washington, DC, where he helped bioscience and technology companies shape federal regulations and policies. Previously, he worked at Louisiana's higher education oversight agency, the Board of Regents, managing the state's STEM (Science, Technology, Engineering, and Mathematics) Advisory Council. As the only hired staff for the council, Dr. Dunn was responsible for leading legislative research and analysis work, strategic partnerships, fundraising, policy recommendations for the state legislature, and planning and executing an inaugural STEM summit. He holds a B.S. in psychology and chemistry from Xavier University of Louisiana and a Ph.D. in neurobiology from Louisiana State University.

Dominic LoBuglio is a senior program assistant in the U.S. Science and Innovation Policy Theme at the National Academies of Sciences, Engineering, and Medicine. In addition to the policy theme itself, much of his work centers around the Committee on Science, Technology, and Law and its related projects. Prior to coming to the National Academies in 2019, Mr. LoBuglio developed outreach and science education programs within the fundraising department of the Natural History Museum of Los Angeles County. Previously, he also worked in the science and technology division at the Los Angeles office of the Japan External Trade Organization, a section of the Japanese government's Ministry of Economy, Trade, and Industry. Mr. LoBuglio holds a B.A. in Japanese language and culture from the University of California, Santa Barbara.

Sarah Carter, Ph.D., is principal at Science Policy Consulting, LLC, where she focuses on societal and policy implications of emerging biotechnologies. In addition to human neural organoids, transplants, and chimeras, she is currently focused on the future of the advanced biotechnologies industry, synthetic biology and DNA sequence screening, and international norms. Previously, Dr. Carter worked in the Policy Center of the J. Craig Venter Institute, where she led influential projects on the accelerating pace of synthetic biology and the challenges it creates for policy makers. In 2009–2010, she was a policy analyst at the White House Office of Science and Technology Policy. Dr. Carter is also a former Science and Technology Policy Fellow with the American Association for the Advancement of Science and a former Mirzayan Fellow of the National Academies. She earned a B.A. in biology from Duke University and a Ph.D. in neuroscience from the University of California, San Francisco.

Appendix B

Committee Meeting Agendas

Meeting 1

June 1, 2020

OPEN SESSION

12:30pm	Welcome, Introductions, and Meeting Overview
	Committee Co-Chairs: **Bernard Lo**, The Greenwall Foundation (retired) **Joshua Sanes**, Harvard University
12:40 pm	Charge to Committee
	Speaker: **Carrie Wolinetz**, National Institutes of Health
1:30 pm	Neural Organoids: The State of the Science
	Speaker: **Arnold Kriegstein**, University of California, San Francisco
1:50 pm	Q&A with Committee

2:30 pm	Neural Chimeras: The State of the Science
	Speaker: **Steven Goldman**, University of Rochester Medical Center
2:50 pm	Q&A with Committee
3:30 pm	Adjourn to Closed Session

June 2, 2020

OPEN SESSION

12:00 pm	Welcome
	Committee Co-Chairs: **Bernard Lo**, The Greenwall Foundation (retired) **Joshua Sanes**, Harvard University
12:05 pm	The Ethics of Neural Organoid and Chimera Research
	Speaker: **Nita Farahany**, Duke University School of Law
12:25 pm	Q&A with Committee
1:00 pm	The Regulatory Landscape for Neural Organoid and Chimera Research
	Speaker: **I. Glenn Cohen**, Harvard Law School
1:20 pm	Q&A with Committee
2:00 pm	Adjourn to Closed Session

Meeting 2
July 15, 2020

3:00 pm	Sponsor Perspective
	Speaker: **Steven E. Hyman**, Harvard University and Board Chair, Dana Foundation
3:10 pm	Discussion with Committee
3:30 pm	Improving Scientific Communication about Complex Concepts
	Speaker: **Kathleen Hall Jamieson**, University of Pennsylvania
3:40 pm	Discussion with Committee
4:00	Adjourn to Closed Session

Meeting 3
August 10, 2020

OPEN SESSION

Framing Questions for Meeting Discussions:

- How would researchers define or identify enhanced or human awareness in a chimeric animal?
- Do research animals with enhanced capabilities require different treatment compared to typical animal models? What are appropriate disposal mechanisms for such models?
- How large or complex would the ex vivo brain organoids need to be to attain enhanced or human awareness?

1:00 pm Welcome, Introductions, and Meeting Overview

Committee Co-Chairs:
Bernard Lo, The Greenwall Foundation (retired)
Joshua Sanes, Harvard University

1:05 pm	Consciousness and Awareness
	Speakers: **Anil Seth**, University of Sussex **Christof Koch**, Allen Institute for Brain Science **Eva Jablonka**, Tel-Aviv University
1:45 pm	Q&A with Committee
2:30 pm	Break
2:45 pm	Understanding and Measuring Consciousness in Animals
	Speakers: **David DeGrazia**, George Washington University **Frans B. M. de Waal**, Emory University
3:15 pm	Q&A with Committee
4:00 pm	States of Consciousness in Humans
	Speakers: **Emery Brown**, Massachusetts Institute of Technology **Brian Edlow**, Massachusetts General Hospital
4:30 pm	Q&A with Committee
5:30 pm	Adjourn

August 11, 2020

OPEN SESSION

12:00 pm	Welcome
	Committee Co-Chairs: **Bernard Lo**, The Greenwall Foundation (retired) **Joshua Sanes**, Harvard University
12:05 pm	Understanding and Measuring Pain in Animals
	Speakers: **Megan Albertelli**, Stanford University **Allan Basbaum**, University of California, San Francisco

APPENDIX B

12:35 pm	Q&A with Committee
1:15 pm	Break / Adjourn to Closed Session

Meeting 4
September 25, 2020

OPEN SESSION

12:00 pm	Welcome
	Committee Co-Chairs: **Bernard Lo**, The Greenwall Foundation (retired) **Joshua Sanes**, Harvard University
12:10 pm	Neural Chimeras and Organoids and Other Human Organoids: Research Methods and Materials
	Speakers: **Bjoern Schwer**, University of California, San Francisco **Sergiu Pasca**, Stanford University **Gordana Vunjak-Novakovic**, Columbia University
1:15 pm	Discussion with Committee
2:00 pm	Break
2:15 pm	Nonhuman Primate Neural Research
	Speakers: **Mu-Ming Poo**, Institute of Neuroscience of the Chinese Academy of Sciences **Guoping Feng**, Massachusetts Institute of Technology
3:00 pm	Discussion with Committee
4:00 pm	Adjourn to Closed Session

Meeting 5
October 29, 2020

OPEN SESSION

12:00 pm	Welcome
	Committee Co-Chairs: **Bernard Lo**, The Greenwall Foundation (retired) **Joshua Sanes**, Harvard University
12:15 pm	Communication and Engagement with the Public
	Speakers: **Dietram Scheufele**, University of Wisconsin–Madison **Brad Margus**, Cerevance **Evelynn Hammonds**, Harvard University
1:00 pm	Q&A with Committee
2:00 pm	Break
2:15 pm	Religious Perspectives, Pt. 1
	Speakers: **Sarra Tlili**, University of Florida **John Loike**, Columbia University
2:45 pm	Q&A with Committee
3:30 pm	Break and Adjourn to Closed Session

October 30, 2020

OPEN SESSION

1:00 pm	Welcome
	Committee Co-Chairs: **Bernard Lo**, The Greenwall Foundation (retired) **Joshua Sanes**, Harvard University

1:05 pm	Religious Perspectives, Pt. 2
	Speaker: **Charles Camosy**, Fordham University
1:20 pm	Q&A with Committee
2:00 pm	Break
2:15 pm	Animal Welfare
	Speakers: **Margaret Landi**, GlaxoSmithKline **Joyce Tischler**, Lewis & Clark Law School
2:45 pm	Q&A with Committee
3:30 pm	Break and Adjourn to Closed Session

Meeting 6
November 13, 2020

OPEN SESSION

12:00 pm	Welcome
	Committee Co-Chairs: **Bernard Lo**, The Greenwall Foundation (retired) **Joshua Sanes**, Harvard University
12:05 pm	Forthcoming ISSCR Guidelines
	Speaker: **Insoo Hyun**, Case Western Reserve University
12:25 pm	Discussion with Committee
1:00 pm	Public Engagement and International Governance
	Speaker: **Robin Lovell-Badge**, The Francis Crick Institute

1:20 pm	Discussion with Committee
1:55 pm	Break and Adjourn to Closed Session
3:00 pm	Adjourn to Open Session

OPEN SESSION

3:00 pm	Mechanism for Governance: NeXTRAC
	Speaker: **Margaret Foster Riley**, University of Virginia School of Law
3:20 pm	Discussion with Committee
4:00 pm	International Regulation of Neural Organoids and Chimeras
	Speakers: **Valerie Bonham**, Ropes & Gray LLP **Mark Barnes**, Ropes & Gray LLP
4:30 pm	Discussion with Committee
5:00 pm	Adjourn to Closed Session

Meeting 7
December 15, 2020

OPEN SESSION

2:00 pm	Religious Perspectives, Pt. 3
	Moderator: **Bernard Lo**, The Greenwall Foundation (retired)
	Speaker: **James Peterson**, Roanoke College
2:15 pm	Q&A with Committee
3:00 pm	Adjourn to Closed Session